Recent Advances in
THIN-LAYER
CHROMATOGRAPHY

Recent Advances in
THIN-LAYER
CHROMATOGRAPHY

Edited by

F. A. A. Dallas
Glaxo Group Research Limited
Ware, United Kingdom

H. Read
BP Research Centre
Sunbury-on-Thames, United Kingdom

R. J. Ruane and I. D. Wilson
ICI Pharmaceuticals Division
Macclesfield, United Kingdom

PLENUM PRESS • NEW YORK AND LONDON

Library of Congress Cataloging in Publication Data

Chromatographic Society International Symposium on Thin-Layer Chromatography
(1987: Brighton, East Sussex)
  Recent advances in thin-layer chromatography.

  "Proceedings of the Chromatographic Society International Symposium on Thin-
Layer Chromatography, held March 11–12, 1987, in Brighton, United Kingdom"—CIP
copr. p.
  Bibliography: p.
  Includes index.
  1. Thin layer chromatography—Congresses. I. Dallas, F. A. A. II. Chromatographic
Society. III. Title.
QD79.C8C47 1987   543′.08956   88-17880
ISBN 0-306-42934-9

Proceedings of the Chromatographic Society International Symposium on Thin-Layer
Chromatography, held March 11–12, 1987, in Brighton, United Kingdom

© 1988 Plenum Press, New York
A Division of Plenum Publishing Corporation
233 Spring Street, New York, N.Y. 10013

PREFACE

For many years TLC has suffered from the image of being a low
sensitivity, low resolution, non-quantitative technique, suitable for
chemists, but not a tool for real chromatographers. Whilst perhaps true
in the past this attitude no longer reflects the capabilities of modern
instrumentalized TLC in all its many forms. This volume represents the
proceedings of a meeting in Brighton in 1987 which formed part of a
continuing series of one and two day events on TLC organized by the
Chromatographic Society either alone or, like this one, in conjunction with
other learned bodies. These meetings are designed to keep chromatographers
up to date with the latest developments and help promote a more positive
image of TLC.

Ian Wilson

November 1987

CONTENTS

THE CHROMATOGRAPHIC SOCIETY

The Chromatographic society is the only international organization devoted to the promotion of, and the exchange of information on, all aspects of chromatography and related techniques.

With the introduction of gas chromatography in 1952, the Hydrocarbon Chemistry Panel of the Hydrocarbon Research Group of the Institute of Petroleum, recognizing the potential of this new technique, set up a Committee under Dr. S. F. Birch to organize a Symposium on 'Vapor Phase Chromatography' which was held in London in June 1956. Almost 400 delegates attended this meeting and success exceeded all expectation. It was immediately apparent that there was a need for an organized forum to afford discussion of development and application of the method and, by the end of the year, the Gas Chromatography Discussion Group had been formed under the Chairmanship of Dr. A. T. James with D. H. Desty as Secretary. Membership of this Group was originally by invitation only but, in deference to popular demand, the Group was opened to all willing to pay the modest subscription of one guinea and in 1957 A.J.P. Martin, Nobel Laureate, was elected inaugural Chairman of the newly-expanded Discussion Group.

In 1958 a second Symposium was organized, this time in conjunction with the Dutch Chemical Society, and since that memorable meeting in Amsterdam the Group, now Society, has maintained close contact with kindred bodies in other countries, particularly France (Groupement pour l'Avancement des Methodes Spectroscopiques et Physico-chimiques d'Analyse) and Germany (Arbeitskreis Chromatographie der Gesellschaft Deutscher Chemiker) as well as interested parties in Eire, Italy, The Netherlands, Scandinavia, Spain and Switzerland. As a result Chromatography Symposia, in association with Instrument Exhibitions, have been held biennially in Amsterdam, Edinburgh, Hamburg, Brighton, Rome, Copenhagen, Dublin, Montreux, Barcelona, Birmingham, Baden-Baden, Cannes, London Nurnburg and Paris.

In 1958 'Gas Chromatography Abstracts' was introduced in journal format under the Editorship of C.E.H. Knapman; first published by Butterworths, then by the Institute of Petroleum, it now appears as 'Gas and Liquid Chromatography Abstracts' produced by Elsevier Applied Science Publishers and is of international status – abstracts, covering all aspects of chromatography, are collected by Members from over 200 sources and collated by the Editor Mr. E. R. Adlard assisted by Dr. P. S. Sewell.

Links with the Institute of Petroleum were severed at the end of 1972 and the Group established a Secretariat at Trent Polytechnic in Nottingham, Professor Ralph Stock playing a prominent part in the establishment of the Group as an independent body. At the same time, in recognition of expanding horizons, the name of the organization was changed to the Chromatography Discussion Group.

In 1978, the 'Father' of Partition Chromatography, Professor A. J. P. Martin was both honoured and commemorated by the institution of the Martin Award which is designed as testimony of distinguished contribution to the advancement of chromatography. Recipients of the award include:-

E.R. Adlard	Prof. E. Bayer
Prof. L.S. Ettre	Prof. G. Guiochon
Dr. C.E.R. Jones	C.E.H. Knapman
Prof. J.H. Knox	Prof. E. Kovats
Prof. A. Liberti	Dr. C.S.G. Phillips
Dr. G. Schomburg	Dr. R.P.W. Scott
Prof. R. Stock	Dr. G.A.P. Tuey

The Group celebrated its Silver Jubilee in 1982 with the 14th International Symposium held, appropriately, in London. To commemorate that event the Jubilee Medal was struck as means of recognising significant contributions by younger workers in the field. Then, the recipients were Dr. K. Grob Jr. and Dr. R. Tijssen, while in 1984 the Medal was awarded to Dr. P. G. Simmonds.

In 1984 the name was once again changed, this time to THE CHROMATOGRAPHIC SOCIETY, which title was believed to be more in keeping with the role of a learned society having an international membership of some 1,000 scientists drawn from more than 40 countries. At that time, the Executive Committee instituted Conference and Travel Bursaries in order to assist Members wishing to contribute to, or attend major meetings throughout the world.

The Society is run by an Executive Committee elected by its Members, in addition to the international symposia, seven or eight one-day meetings covering a wide range of subjects are organized annually. One of these meetings, the Spring Symposium, is coupled with the Society's Annual General Meeting when, in addition to electing the Society's Executive Committee, Members have the opportunity to express their views on the Society's activities and offer suggestions for future policy.

Regular training courses in all aspects of chromatography are run in conjunction with the Robens Institute of the University of Surrey and it is hoped that this particular service will eventually include advanced and highly specialised instruction.

Reports of the Society's activities, in addition to other items of interest to its members (including detailed summaries of all papers presented at its meetings), are given in the Chromatographic Society Bulletin which is produced quarterly under the editorship of I.W. Davies.

At the time of writing three grades of membership are offered:-

Membership with Abstracts	£20.00 per year
Membership	£11.00 per year
Student Membership (includes Abstracts)	£6.00 per year

Members receive the Bulletin free of charge, benefit from concessionary Registration Fees for all Meetings and Training Courses and are, of course, eligible to apply for Travel and/or Conference Bursaries.

For further information please write to:-

Mrs. J. Challis
Executive Secretary
THE CHROMATOGRAPHIC SOCIETY
Trent Polytechnic
Burton Street
Nottingham NG1 4BU
United Kingdom.

CONTEMPORARY THIN-LAYER CHROMATOGRAPHY: AN INTRODUCTION

Ian D. Wilson

Department of Safety of Medicines
ICI Pharmaceuticals Division, Mereside
Alderley Park, Macclesfield, Cheshire SK10 4TG, UK

SUMMARY

Thin-layer chromatography (TLC) is at last beginning to overcome the poor image from which it has suffered in the past. With the development of high performance TLC plates, the introduction of new stationary phases and the instrumentalization of virtually all aspects of the technique TLC has been transformed into a modern sensitive and high performance analytical method. Current advances in TLC are briefly reviewed including developments in stationary phases, techniques of development and methods of detection.

INTRODUCTION

Thin-layer chromatography (TLC), which came into general usage following the pioneering work of Stahl has now been practised for over 40 years. Despite the introduction of other chromatographic techniques, particularly high performance liquid chromatography (HPLC) the use of TLC has not declined noticeably and currently shows signs of a resurgence in popularity led by the introduction of new stationary phases and greatly improved instrumentation. Thus, even though it is highly improbable that TLC will ever replace HPLC as the major chromatographic method it also seems increasingly unlikely that the technique will ever fall into disuse, in stark contrast to paper chromatography which has now attained the status of a lost art.

TLC is probably the most accessible of all chromatographic methods requiring, at its most basic, only the plate itself, solvent and a suitable container to place them both in for development. Evaluation of the plate may then be accomplished with the aid of nothing more sophisticated than the human eye, perhaps aided by using any one of the many hundreds of spray reagents (of varying degrees of specificity) which have been developed since the technique was first described.

This type of TLC is essentially simple, robust, has a large sample capacity, is rapid, and makes only modest demands on equipment, resources and trained personnel. Indeed for qualitative or semi-quantitative analysis it is difficult to envisage a better method than TLC. Perversely, it is probably because it can be performed so simply that TLC has acquired

1

the stigma of being a low resolution method, of poor sensitivity, and incapable of being applied to the problem of providing accurate, precise and specific methods. Such a view is demonstrably incorrect and can be likened to dismissing the possibility of obtaining sensitive and quantitative results from HPLC based on experiences gained with open column chromatography. Clearly when used badly even instrumentalized TLC gives poor results, and it is certainly the case that the development of instrumentation for TLC and high performance (HP) TLC has lagged behind that of other chromatographic techniques. However, this situation is being remedied, and the difference between modern instrumentalized HPTLC and the older, more basic, TLC methods is indeed as large as that which exists between HPLC and the open columns techniques which preceeded it.

No one would claim that the new TLC is superior to HPLC or GLC in all applications (which is patently absurd) however, there are many circumstances where it offers a viable alternative. Indeed there are often occasions when TLC may offer significant advantages over other techniques. For example, in cases where concentrations in the sample are high, high sample throughput is required and the sample causes a rapid deterioration in the performance of HPLC or GLC columns then TLC becomes the method of choice.

TLC Plates

Traditionally TLC has been performed using a limited range of stationary phases (silica gel, alumina, cellulose, kieselghur and polyamide) coated onto glass, plastic or aluminium foil. Of all the materials used for TLC, silica gel is by far the most popular and is likely to remain so for the foreseeable future. However, within the last decade, due no doubt to the advances in the preparation of bonded silicas for HPLC, a range of alkyl bonded silica TLC plates have been introduced. These include C_{18}, C_{12}, C_8, C_2, aminopropyl, diphenyl and cyanopropyl bonded plates, as well as a type of plate coated with a chiral complexing agent designed for the separation of amino acid enantiomers and similar compounds (the "chiral plate" from Machery-Nagel)[1] (see also Rausch, this vol.).

Bonded Phases

The range of bonded phases is still quite limited compared to those available for HPLC but is continually being expanded as more types are introduced into use in HPLC. The introduction of these bonded silicas has led to a renewed interest in reversed-phase (RP) TLC, but for a number of reasons it is unlikely that this mode of chromatography will become as popular in TLC as it is in HPLC. This is primarily because normal phase (NP) TLC suffers from few of the problems afflicting NP-HPLC on silica gel (i.e. poor reproducibility, rapid loss of performance, restricted range of sample types resulting in the need to exclude aqueous samples). The reasons for this are not hard to find as the bulk of the problem of poor reproducibility in NP-HPLC results from the activation or deactivation of the silica gel in the column by the continuous flow of the mobile phase. This can, over a period of time, cause changes in peak shape and retention. In HPLC this problem has been overcome by using bonded silicas and reversed-phase chromatography. In contrast, in TLC where the plate is only used once, it is of no importance that its chromatographic properties may have changed during the run. Furthermore, as the solvent in which the sample is applied is removed prior to the development of the plate it too is unlikely to be the cause of major chromatographic problems. Aqueous samples such as urine, bile and plasma can therefore be applied to silica TLC plates without difficulty. Additional reasons for the likely continued use of NP-TLC are some practical difficulties which limit the application of RP-TLC. The major limitation being the intensely hydrophobic nature of the bulk of commercially available C_{18}, C_8 and C_2 bonded HPTLC plates. This makes the use of mobile phases containing "large" amounts of water (greater than ~40%) either impractical or only possible with very long development times (in excess of 1 or 2 hours). Certain of the bonded plates can be used with solvents containing a high proportion of water (up to 100%) in the solvent including a C_{12} plate from Antec and a C_{18} plate from E. Merck. However, both of these types of plate are only available as TLC, rather than HPTLC plates. Recently however a fully wettable C_{18} bonded HPTLC has been introduced by Merck which can also be used without restrictions on the solvent composition. As well as this new C_{18} phase the cyanopropyl and aminopropyl HPTLC plates now available can also be used with water rich mobile phases (see Fischer et. al., this vol.).

A particular advantage which we have found when using RP-TLC is the very wide range over which a linear relationship between R and the eluotropic strength of the solvent often exists. This makes method development relatively easy, especially as minor variations (1 or 2%) in solvent composition do not have major effects on R_F. This observation contrasts markedly with our experiences with silica where, because the linear range is narrower and the slope steeper, very small changes in solvent composition can have dramatic effects of R_F and spot shape.

Although there are, at first sight, many similarities between RP-HPLC and RP-TLC there are pitfalls in attempting to transfer expertise gained using one technique to the other. Perhaps the most obvious difference in our hands is the relatively minor importance of the control of solvent pH in RP-TLC. Thus, in cases where the RP-HPLC method for an acidic drug required a solvent pH of ~2 we found that with RP-TLC changing the pH between 2 and 9 had no effect on factors such as spot shape and R_F. Similarly with ion-pair RP-TLC, pH can be a much less important factor in determining R_F than it is for retention in RP-HPLC (although this depends to some extent on the structure of the IP-reagent[2-4]. For example, in the case of symmetrical compounds such as tetramethyl or tetra-n-butylammonium bromide the pH of the solvent had no effect on the subsequent R of the acidic compounds with which they ion-pair. However, with unsymmetrical compounds such as cetrimide (cetyltrimethylammonium bromide) the pH of the solvent can be an important factor controlling R_F. As yet we have been unable to detect an effect of solvent pH on R_F with sulphonic acid (e.g. heptane-sulphonic acid) ion-pair reagents (Ruane and Wilson, unpublished observations). In many ways these results are rather surprising, given the importance of pH in IP-HPLC, and deserve further investigation.

Whilst NP-TLC is probably the method of first choice, we have found circumstances, particularly in the case of compounds of limited stability on silica gel, where RP-TLC on C_{18} bonded and C_{12} bonded plates[5] has proved to be superior.

High-Performance Thin-Layer Chromatography (HPTLC)

Another major development in the elevation of TLC from a qualitative or semi-quantitative technique into a sensitive and flexible quantitative system was the introduction of high performance TLC plates. HPTLC differs from conventional TLC in a number of ways but mainly in the size of the particles used in the manufacture of the plates and in the need for a much more precise and instrumentalized approach in order to obtain the best results from them. Thus, conventional TLC plates are generally about 0.10 to 0.25 mm thick and are formed from silica with a mean particle size of ~20 μm and a wide particle size distribution. Development distances are usually in the order of 15 to 17 cm and the run time is often measured in periods of hours rather than minutes. For HPTLC the particle size is usually between 5 and 10 μm with much tighter control over the size distribution. The layers produced for HPTLC are usually 100–250 μm thick with separations usually accomplished quite rapidly using development distances of 5 to 10 cm. The small particle size and more uniform nature of the silica gel results in much greater chromatographic efficiency than found in ordinary TLC and enables the same separations to be achieved much more rapidly.

A large number of claims have been made for the advantage of HPTLC over TLC including, amongst others, increased resolution, greater sensitivity, better reproducibility, greater numbers of sample per plate, all combined with performance approaching that of HPLC. All of these may be true; however, these advantages have not been obtained without cost. In particular the simplicity and robustness of ordinary TLC (which make it almost foolproof) are not so evident in HPTLC where all stages from the spotting of the sample, through chromatography, and evaluation all require much greater control and the involvement of instrumentation such as auto-spotters and development chambers. A final note of caution must be extended to include the products themselves. Most TLC plate manufacturers now produce "HPTLC" plates, but the quality of some of these leaves much to be desired and care is required in the selection of these plates if true HPTLC is to be performed.

Development Techniques

As stated in the introduction, in the beginning TLC was performed simply by placing the plate in a glass tank containing an appropriate amount of solvent which was then allowed to migrate the required distance needed to obtain the desired separation. There are currently in existence a large variety of development techniques devised in order to improve upon the type of separation afforded by the basic TLC technique. These methods include continuous development, multiple development and its instrumentalized variants of programmed multiple development (PMD)[6] and automated multiple development (AMD)[7], continuous multiple development (which combines the continuous and multiple development techniques),[8] circular (or radial) and anti-circular development[9], over-pressurized TLC[10], two dimensional TLC,[11] two-phase two-dimensional TLC,[12] triangular development[13], and centrifugal development[14]. The essential features of some of these systems are described below.

In continuous development the fact that the migration velocity of the mobile phase is inversely proportional to the square of the distance travelled is exploited. The solvent is allowed to travel a short distance up the plate at which point it is continuously evaporated, thus permitting the separation to be achieved more rapidly than in ordinary development.

For multiple development and its associated instrumentalized techniques (PMD and AMD) the TLC plate is repeatedly redeveloped (with or without changing the composition of the solvent system). This can allow components to be separated a few at a time by using different solvent systems at each stage. Alternatively by using the same solvent and allowing the solvent front to advance a little further at each stage increased resolution between spots can be achieved. The latter technique has the added advantage that with each development a certain amount of spot reconcentration occurs giving sharper signals and thus better sensitivity. These techniques are certainly capable of producing impressive separations, although this must be paid for in terms of increased analysis times and the cost of the equipment. An example of the separation obtained for some polyhydroxysteroids using "manual" multiple development and the AMD technique is given in Figure 1.

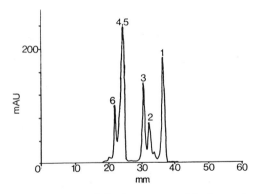

Fig. 1. Separation of some polyhydroxysteroids by automated multiple
development on silica gel HPTLC plates (25 developments using
methanol-dichloromethane 7.5:95.5).
Key: 1, polypodine B 2-cinnamate; 2, ponasterone A; 3, ponasterone
C; 4, ecdysone; 5, polypodine B; 6, makisterone A.

    With circular development the solvent is fed into the center of the
plate and migrates out towards the edges. Conversely, with anti-circular
development the solvent migrates from the edges of the plate towards the
center. Various advantages are claimed for these modes of development and
Kaiser in a comparison of them found anticircular TLC to give the best
results in terms of sensitivity, number of samples per plate, speed of
analysis and lowest solvent use[9]. Conventional TLC was ranked second
with circular TLC the poorest except for the separation number (the number
of components which could be resolved) where it was superior to both anticircular and conventional TLC, (see also the article by Traitler and
Studer, this vol.).

    Overpressurized TLC (OPTLC or OPLC) is a relatively new technique
whereby the plate is covered by a flexible membrane held in place by an
external pressure (see also Mincsovics, this vol.). The solvent is then
pumped into the layer in order to effect a separation, thus providing a
system which is intermediate in its properties between HPLC and TLC (a sort
of planar column chromatography!).

    Another innovation is centrifugal layer chromatography (CLC) where
solvent is fed into the center of a rotating TLC plate. The solvent migrates more rapidly than in conventional TLC driven by centrifugal force as
well as capillary action. Devices for CLC are available for both analytical and preparative scale chromatography and it will be interesting to see
how the technique evolves (see also Nyiredy, Dallenbach-Toelke and Sticher,
this vol.).

Detection and Quantification

    In the basic TLC technique, detection is based on the human eye aided
by a vast array of selective spray reagents and the use of plates impregnated with fluorescent indicators which allow compounds to be detected by
fluorescence quenching. For quantitative evaluation, especially in HPTLC,
a range of TLC UV/visible scanners are available which are capable of
operating in any one of several modes. Thus scanners are available which
can measure absorbance, fluorescence and fluorescence quenching and many
are capable of obtaining the spectra of the individual spots in situ (see
Poole, Poole and Dean, this vol.). Apart from this type of detector many
other systems have been described including the use of a video camera and

5

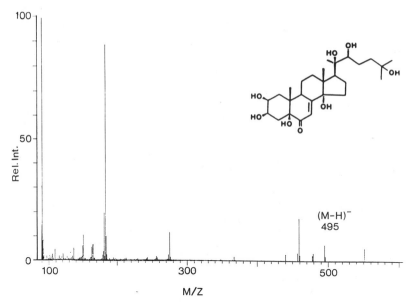

Fig. 2. Mass spectrum of polypodine B (see insert for structure) using
fast atom bombardment (-ve, xenon) obtained directly from a silica
gel HPTLC plate.

computer based image processing system as an alternative to scanning densitometry[15]. In addition, other spectroscopic techniques have been
applied to TLC including infra red[16] and mass spectrometry (both on and
off line)[17-19]. Most of these applications of TLC-MS are now based on
the use of fast atom bombardment (FAB) from silica gel. (See Figure 2 for
an example). However, it is possible to use less sophisticated methods of
ionization, such as electron impact (EI) with stationary phases such as
polyamide or cellulose. Obviously as a tool for identification the combination of TLC with mass-spectrometry has many of the same advantages as
GC or HPLC-MS without the need to have a complicated interface between
chromatography and spectrometer. For TLC-MS the appropriate area of silica
is simply removed from the plate and placed on the probe of the mass spectrometer. Yet another type of detection system is provided by the Iatroscan device where chromatography is performed on silica gel coated quartz
rods with detection by a flame ionization detector. In another field, that
of the TLC analysis of radioactive substances on TLC plates, the introduction of a new type of detector (the so called linear analyzer) has re-
volutionized detection and quantification, with as little as 100 dpm of
radioactive carbon 14 detectable by such instruments[20].

Thus, over the last decade considerable innovation has taken place in
the area of instrumental TLC and HPTLC greatly increasing the potential of
the technique. However, it must be continually emphasized that, in order
to get the best results using these quantitative techniques much more
control is needed at all stages of sample application and chromatography.
In the case of sample application the autospotters currently available can
apply as little as 50 µl with a precision of about 1% as spots, whilst the
Linomat III (Camag) can apply from 2 to 99 µl as a streak.

CONCLUSIONS

Despite a slow start compared to HPLC and GLC the last decade has seen
a rapid evolution in the potential of TLC. At one extreme there remains

the basic technique, robust, simple and cheap, ideal for rapid qualitative results. At the other extreme are a range of instrumentalized variants on the general theme of TLC capable of giving good resolution combined with reliable, precise and accurate quantitative results very rapidly and with the possibility of a very high sample throughput. Even more encouraging is the fact that TLC once again appears to be attracting innovative researchers who will continue to advance the capabilities of the technique and not let it stagnate as happened in the past.

It is still unlikely that TLC, in any of its forms, will ever displace HPLC and GLC from their current positions, especially given the huge investments that have been made in these techniques. However it is now the case that for many applications TLC represents an alternative to these other systems. Certainly it is no longer possible to say about TLC that it is a low resolution, semi-qualitative or quantitative technique, with poor sensitivity, useful for chemists, but not a real quantitative tool for analysts and chromatographers. Most of the steps in quantitative TLC can, or have been, automated and it ought not to be difficult to automate the whole procedure, especially with the current advances in laboratory robotics. Such developments can only make the use of TLC an even more attractive proposition.

REFERENCES

1. K. Günther, J. Martens, and M. Schickendanz, Angew.Chem.Int.Ed.Engl., 23:506 (1984).
2. S. Lewis and I. D. Wilson, J.Chromatogr., 312:133 (1984).
3. I. D. Wilson, J.Chromatogr., 354:99 (1986).
4. J. A. Troke and I. D. Wilson, J.Chromatogr., 360:236 (1986).
5. I. D. Wilson, J.Pharm.Biomed.Anal., 1:219 (1983).
6. J. A. Perry and L. J. Glunz, J.Chromatogr.Sci., 11:447 (1973).
7. K. D. Burger and H. Tengler, in: R. E. Kaiser, (ed.), Planar Chromatography 1, Dr Alfred Heuthig Verlag, Heidelberg, p.143 (1986).
8. K. W. Lee, C. F. Poole and A. Zlatkis, in: W. Bertsch, S. Hara, R. E. Kaiser and A. Zlatkis, (eds.), "Instrumental HPTLC," Dr Alfred Heuthig Verlag, Heidelberg, p.245 (1980).
9. R. E. Kaiser, in: A. Zlatkis and R. E. Kaiser, (eds.), "HPTLC - High Performance Thin Layer Chromatography," Elsevier/North Holland Biomedical Press, Amsterdam, p.73. (1977).
10. Z. Lengyl, E. Tyihák and E. Mincsovics, J.Liq.Chromatogr., 5:1541 (1981).
11. M. Azkaria, M.-F. Gonnord, and G. Guiochon, J.Chromatogr., 271:127 (1983).
12. H. J. Issaq, J.Liq.Chromatogr., 3:841 (1980).
13. H. J. Issaq, J.Liq.Chromatogr., 3:789 (1980).
14. S. Z. Nyiredi, C. A. J. Erdelmeier, and O. Sticher, in: R. E. Kaiser (ed.), "Planar Chromatography 1, Dr Alfred Heuthig Verlag, Heidelberg, p. 119 (1986).
15. R. M. Belchamber, H. Read and D. M. Roberts, in: R. E. Kaiser, "Planar Chromatography 1, Dr Alfred Heuthig Verlag, Heidelberg, p. 207 (1986).
16. G. E. Zuber, R. J. Warren, P. P. Begosh, and E. L. O'Donnell, Anal. Chem., 56:2935 (1984).
17. T. T. Change, J. O. Lay Jnr., and R. J. Francel, Anal.Chem., 56:111 (1984).
18. L. Ramaley, M.-A. Vaughan, and W. D. Jamieson, Anal.Chem., 57:353 (1985).
19. K. J. Bare, and H. Read, The Analyst, 112:433 (1987).

20. H. Filthuth, in: D. M. Wieland, M. C. Tobes, and T. J. Mangner, (eds.), "Analytical and Chromatographic Techniques in Radiopharmaceutical Chemistry," Spring-Verlag, New York, p. 79 (1986).

INSTRUMENTATION

QUANTITATIVE METHODS IN THIN-LAYER CHROMATOGRAPHY

Colin F. Poole*, Salwa K. Poole, and Thomas A. Dean

Department of Chemistry
Wayne State University
Detroit, Michigan 48202, USA

SUMMARY

Physical, chemical and instrumental sources of error in quantitative thin-layer chromatography using slit-scanning densitometry are identified, and where possible, practical solutions for their control are indicated. Mathematical transformations of non-linear calibration data are identified as an additional source of error that can be avoided by using nonlinear regression models. In addition, some alternative techniques to quantification by slit-scanning densitometry are considered and their future assessed. From among these, image analyzers and hyphenated techniques such as TLC-SIMS and TLC-SERS, which can provide structural information from TLC spots for identification purposes, are highlighted as being likely to become more important in the near future.

INTRODUCTION

Many changes have occurred in the practice of thin-layer chromatography (TLC) in the last ten years. Methods of sample application, plate materials, and development strategies have been optimized to improve the performance and speed of thin-layer separations[1-5]. Analysts involved in developing these new technologies have variously called the technique "high performance", "instrumental", or "modern" thin-layer chromatography to distance themselves from the body of scientists who still apply the conventional practices of TLC as developed during the 1950's. Modern TLC is characterized by the optimization of the separation and chromatogram recording process by use of instrumental procedures. This process was readily accepted in column liquid chromatography but mysteriously still meets with resistance when applied to TLC. Thus, we now have a division among thin-layer chromatographers; one group remain convinced that TLC is an elegant method for the qualitative analysis of simple mixtures while the second are equally convinced that TLC can provide much more than qualitative information and need not be restricted to the analysis of simple mixtures. Quantification in modern TLC is both accurate and precise and can be applied reliably to problems in major, minor, and trace component analysis. Of equal importance, quantification can be automated, freeing the analyst to perform other tasks.

11

In this chapter we will discuss some of the practical problems that effect the quality of quantitative data in thin-layer chromatography. Where problems still remain we will try and cast our vision forward to touch on those changes in quantitative methods that might be anticipated to occur in the next decade of progress in modern TLC. We will not discuss individual devices for quantitative TLC or the theoretical basis for quantification using optical devices as these aspects are adequately reviewed elsewhere[5-11]. Our aim is to provide some insight into the practice of quantification in TLC, in its broadest sense, for the practicing chromatographer.

SCANNING DENSITOMETRY

We were all born with two very poor detectors for TLC. The eye functions as a logarithmic integrator with a sensitivity of about 1 to 10µg for colored components and a degree of precision rarely better than ± 10 to 30%. The eye is too inaccurate a device to determine correctly either position or concentration data for sample components. Likewise, excising developed spots from the plate followed by solvent elution and spectrophotometric detection is too tedious to be considered an acceptable detection method for a high speed chromatographic technique. It also relies on visual interpretation to decide on the position of zone boundaries as well as being plagued by numerous uncontrolled procedural errors.

Instrumentation for in situ measurement of TLC chromatograms first appeared in the mid-1960s and is absolutely essential for the accurate determination of both spot size and location, for a true measure of resolution, and for rapid, accurate quantification. Modern versions of these early densitometers have evolved into sophisticated, automated, computer-controlled devices. Their data output, whether analog or digital, is in the form of a standard chromatogram obtained by moving the plate at a controlled speed past a fixed measuring transducer. With the exception of radioisotopic detection, the measuring transducer is invariably an optical device and the scanning densitometer can be considered as a spectrophotometer designed to view light reflected or transmitted by an opaque medium instead of a solution.

In situ measurements of substances on TLC plates can be made by a variety of methods: reflectance, transmission, simultaneous reflectance and transmission, fluorescence quenching, and fluorescence. Light striking the plate surface is both transmitted and diffusely scattered by the layer. Light striking a spot on the plate will undergo absorption so that the light transmitted or reflected is diminished in intensity at those wavelengths forming the absorption profile of the spot. The measurement of the signal diminution between the light transmitted or reflected by a blank zone of the plate and a zone containing sample provides the mechanism for quantitative measurements by absorption. For fluorescence measurements the sample beam serves to excite the sample to emit secondary radiation of longer wavelength. Blank zones of the plate are optically dark and the sample zones, can therefore, be considered as point sources of illumination superimposed on this "dark background". From a theoretical and practical point of view this makes quantification much easier as will be outlined later.

The main sources of error in scanning densitometry are the reproducibility of sample application, reproducibility of the chromatographic conditions, reproducibility of positioning the/ spot in the center of the measuring beam, and reproducibility of the measurement[12,13]. The latter is a function of the design of the densitometer and can be determined by repeatedly scanning a single track of the TLC plate without changing any of the experimental variables between scans. It is composed of errors due to the optical measurement, electronic amplification, and the recording device. The measurement error is a function of the sample size, increasing as the detection limit is approached, but should be relatively steady for sample amounts not obviously perturbed by baseline noise. For a properly adjusted instrument values in the range 0.21 to 0.7% are typical. The measurement error should be less than the other three sources of analytical error which, as they are influenced significantly by the conditions selected for the analysis, are more important to our present discussion.

Samples are applied to TLC layers as spots or bands to conform to the demands of minimum size and a homogeneous distribution of sample within the starting zone[8,14]. For fine-particle layer plates, for which desirable starting spot sizes are 1.0mm or less, this corresponds to sample volumes of 100 to 200 nl. For coarse-particle layer plates volumes 5 to 10-fold greater are acceptable. The sample solvent must be a good solvent for the sample to promote quantitative transfer from the sample application device to the layer. It must also be of low viscosity and sufficiently volatile to be easily evaporated from the plate. Further, it must also wet the sorbent layer adequately otherwise penetration of the layer will not occur. It should also be a weak chromatographic solvent for the sample on the sorbent selected for the analysis. Ideally the least retained sample component should have an $R_F<0.1$ if developed in the sample solvent. Generally speaking few problems are encountered in meeting the above criteria when silica gel is used as the sorbent, but for bonded-phase layers, which are not wet very well by aqueous organic solvent mixtures, solvent selection is more problematical. In this case it may be necessary to use methanol, acetonitrile, methylene chloride, or acetone as the sample solvent and to minimize predevelopment of the spot by applying the sample repetitively in small volumes to the layer. Solid-phase transfer devices, such as the contact spotter, allow larger sample volumes to be applied to the plate after solvent removal, but must still conform to the general requirement of providing a starting zone of minimum size, ie., spots $\leq$ 1mm[15,16].

Manual devices for sample application are inappropriate for scanning densitometry. First of all, the starting position of each spot must be known precisely. This is most easily achieved with mechanical devices operating to a precise grid mechanism. The sample must be applied to the layer without disturbing the surface, something that is near to impossible to achieve using manual application. Samples and standards must be applied in the same solvent and identical volumes to insure that identical starting zones are formed. Calibration curves should not be prepared by spotting incremental volumes from a single standard for the above reason. This is illustrated in Figure 1 for two calibration curves prepared by spotting different sample amounts in a constant volume and a constant sample concentration in different volumes. Poor linearity and a non-zero intercept are observed for the sample spotted in a variable volume as well as a considerable offset from the constant volume samples. The sample application error can be effectively eliminated by using an internal standard and maintaining a constant size for the sample starting zone.

The chromatographic error may easily be the most significant error in scanning densitometry and is only reduced by minimizing the variability in the development process. The data pair technique can be used to minimize errors due to migration differences as a result of edge effects, deviations in layer thickness, and non-linear solvent fronts, etc.[17]. The data pair technique is a methods of averaging through internal compensation. Each sample or standard is spotted twice, one spot at the edge of the plate and the other at the center to form one pair, the adjacent spots form the next pair, etc. Each track is scanned twice, an average value taken and then this value is combined by partners and averaged to give the recorded value.

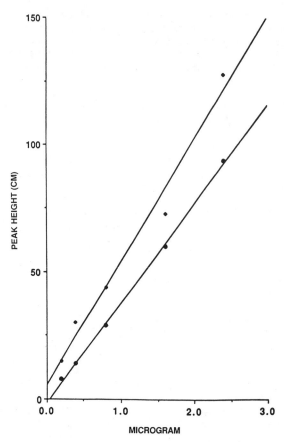

Fig. 1. Calibration curves prepared by spotting a constant volume of
different sample amounts (●) and different volumes of the same
sample amount (◆).

Since the chromatographic error is generally the largest contribution to
the relative standard deviation further improvements in the precision of
TLC analysis will probably only be achieved by improvements to developing
chambers and greater attention being paid to optimizing and standardizing
the development process by the analyst.

   The spot positioning error in the measuring beam can be minimized by
suitable instrument design such as position scanning[9] or zig-zag scanning[19]. In position scanning the spot is detected initially by making
large-search steps in the direction of chromatography, the peak maxima is
then located by making smaller steps, the plate is then moved away from the
established maxima in the direction perpendicular to the direction of the
chromatography and the positioning repeated. This process is continued
until the true peak maxima is located. Each spot, in this way, is
optimally located in the measuring beam independent of the irregularities
in the chromatographic development. This is an automated process performed
under computer control and provided that the sample spot contains a homogeneous distribution of sample within its boundaries then the positioning
error is essentially eliminated. In zig-zag scanning the sample track is
scanned with a rectangular beam of small dimensions with respect to those
of the spot in a saw tooth or square wave pattern by fixing the measuring
beam in one position and mechanically moving the scanning stage in the x-
and y-direction to generate the desired pattern. Under these conditions

the quantitative information obtained is independent of the spot shape and the sample concentration distribution within the spot provided that the measuring beam traverses at least several zones of the spot.

The positioning error will be greatest when manual positioning of each track in the measuring beam during routine analysis is used. This error will also vary with the linearity of the developed track as different zones of each spot further from the origin will be scanned. The use of slit height settings larger than the spot diameter will reduce positioning errors at the expense of some loss in sensitivity. Alternatively, samples can be applied as bands longer than the slit height. The central portion of each band is then scanned. Provided that the sample is distributed homogeneously throughout the band then positioning errors should be very small.

PERFORMANCE CHARACTERISTICS OF SLIT-SCANNING DENSITOMETERS

When assessing the performance of a slit-scanning densitometer the feature of primary concern is the faithfulness with which the densitometer converts the separation into a strip chart (or its electronic equivalent) chromatogram. Here the parameters of interest are the observed resolution, dynamic signal range, and sample detectability, the latter being measured by the signal-to-noise ratio. Experimental variables can also affect these parameters, of which, the most important are the slit dimensions governing the size of the measuring beam, the scan rate, and the total electronic time constant of the instrument and recording device. No standard protocol has been devised to compare the ability of different densitometers to reproduce chromatographic resolution. The influence of experimental variables on the resolution of test chromatograms in the reflectance[19,20] and transmission[20,21] mode for absorption measurements and in the reflectance mode for fluorescence[20,22] measurements has been made. These at least provide a framework by which experimental variables can be optimized to avoid degrading the observed resolution.

Sample detectability is a complex function of both chromatographic and instrumental variables, but unlike the case for resolution, a standard protocol has been developed that is suitable for comparing the performance of individual slit-scanning densitometers as well as enabling detection limits and other sensitivity-dependent parameters to be determined under conditions of know sensitivity[20,23,24]. Azobenzene was selected as a primary standard for the determination using clearly defined chromato- graphic and instrumental parameters, (Table 1). Since there is no simple relationship between signal and spot size, it is necessary to define a single spot size for all measurements. A spot width of 4.0mm was selected as this is in the middle of the range of spot sizes encountered in modern TLC. The slit height (the length of the measuring beam orthogonal to the direction of development) was chosen to be 10% larger than the spot diam- eter. The value of the slit height, or more correctly, the ratio of the slit height to spot diameter, has a profound effect on sensitivity, (Figure 2). When the slit height is large compared to the diameter of the spot, the light flux emanating from blank regions of the plate is large compared to the contribution of absorbed light caused by the presence of the spot. The signal is thus weak. As the slit height is reduced to values close to the spot diameter there is a substantial increase observed in the signal. This arises because the light flux transmitted/reflected by the blank area of the plate is diminished while the amount of light absorbed by the spot remains constant under these circumstances. As the sample concentration across the diameter of the spot is not constant the signal continues to increase as the slit height is reduced to less than the spot diameter. Although a slit setting smaller than the diameter of the spot results in higher sensitivity, the use of small slit dimensions is not practical (unless position or zig-zag scanning is used) because the signal obtained depends on how precisely the measuring beam traverses the exact center of the spot. In general, a 10% excess in the slit height compared to the spot diameter provides adequate signal, ensures that the spot entirely fills the measuring beam, and facilitates manual positioning of the spot with respect to the measuring beam.

Three uses for the standardized protocol can be illustrated (Table 1). Bench mark figures can be provided for the scanning densitometer that can be compared with those of other instruments. Incorporating the protocol into good laboratory practice enables changes in the source intensity to be monitored on a continuous basis. Detection limits for compounds can be determined in a highly reproducible manner and also in such a way that corrections for the operating characteristics of individual instruments are easily made.

In the fluorescence mode a singular difference exists in the relationship between sample detectability and measuring beam dimensions compared to the results discussed above for absorption. There is a linear decrease in signal in going from large to small slit width values (dimensions of the measuring beam in the direction of chromatographic development). As the slit width is decreased, the amount of sample excited during the time the spot is being scanned, is reduced, and consequently fewer molecules are fluorescing and the signal decreases. For changes in slit height, there is

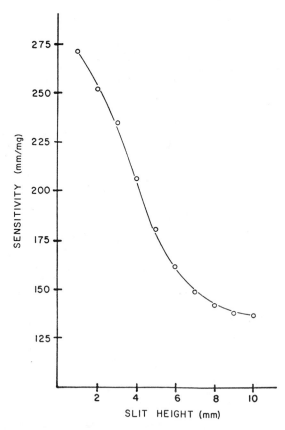

Fig. 2. Relationship between densitometer sensitivity and slit height for a spot of 4.0 mm diameter.

Table 1. Selected Experimental Parameters for Determining Sensitivity and Detectability Values of a Slit-Scanning Densitometer

Parameter	Standard Condition
STANDARD	AZOBENZENE
Concentration (mg/mL)	1.0 (UV)
	5.0 (visible)
Sample Size (nl)	200
Developed spot width (mm)	4.0
Measuring wavelength (nm)	320 (UV)
	430 (visible)
Scan mode	linear
Scan rate (mm/min)	24
Slit width (mm)	0.8
Slit height (mm)	4.4
Sensitivity (mm/ng)	$\dfrac{\text{peak height}}{\text{sample weight}}$
Detectability (ng)	$\dfrac{\text{2 x noise}}{\text{sensitivity}}$

Table 2. Sensitivity and Detectability Data for a Shimadzu CS-910 Scanning Densitometer

1) Operating Mode (new source)	Sensitivity (mm/ng)	Detectability (ng)	
Transmission	0.16 ± 3.8%	4.8 ± 4.0%	
Reflectance	0.15 ± 3.8%	6.0 ± 3.9%	
2) Changes in Source (old source)*			
Transmission	0.14 ± 3.4%	23.7 ± 3.6%	
Reflectance	0.14 ± 3.8%	29.1 ± 4.0%	
3) Accurate Determination of Detection Limits**			
Alprenolol	9.22 ng	13.02	3.26
	8.07 ng	12.89	3.22
	6.92 ng	12.57	3.14
	5.77 ng	12.48	3.12
	4.61 ng	13.67	3.42
	2.31 ng	14.72	3.68
Pamatolol	9.10 ng	10.11	2.53
	7.96 ng	9.92	2.48
	6.83 ng	9.81	2.45
	5.69 ng	10.02	2.51
	4.55 ng	10.99	2.75
Practolol	7.84 ng	16.72	4.18
	6.86 ng	17.73	4.48
	5.88 ng	18.71	4.68

* measurements made with a source determined to be in need of replacement
** amounts shown for beta-blocker antagonists indicates sample size applied to the plate.

a regular increase in signal in going from slit heights less than the spot diameter up to the diameter of the spot, at which point the signal levels off. Thus, to maximize sample detectability for spots of different sizes, large slit height values are preferred; the minimum acceptable value being equivalent to the diameter of the largest spot to be scanned.

SAMPLE CALIBRATION USING SLIT-SCANNING DENSITOMETERS

The relationship between signal response and sample amount is established by calibration for slit-scanning densitometers. In our experience either peak height or peak area measurements can be used with equal reliability. With both measurements it is essential that the substance-spot profile is exactly reproduced for standards and samples. The shape of calibration curves for absorption measurement has caused some concern as these are generally highly non-linear. As opaque media scatter light effectively Beer-Lambert law relationships cannot be expected to apply and an alternative relationship, proposed by Kubelka and Munk, is more appropriate. Solutions to this law may not be exact when applied to thin-layer media, but qualitatively it provides a reasonable description of typical experimental observations. As illustrated in Figure 3, calibration curves are individual in shape, generally comprise a pseudolinear region at low sample concentration curving towards the concentration axis at higher concentrations and eventually reaching some asymptotic value where signal and sample concentration are no longer correlated. The extent of the individual ranges or portions of the calibration curves are frequently very different. In some instances the pseudolinear range may be adequate for most analytical purposes, in others no reasonable linear range may be in existance.

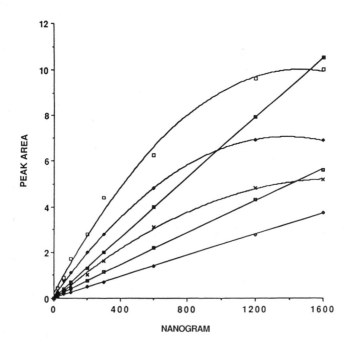

Fig. 3. Some typical calibration curves for various substances measured by absorption in the reflectance mode. Identification; pamatolol (◊), estrone (X), alprenolol (■), diphenylacetylene (♦), azobenzene (□), and practolol (⊞).

Human nature being what it is several methods have been suggested to linearize calibration curves based on either an electronic approximate solution of the Kubelka-Munk equation[11,18] or by simple mathematical transformation techniques using, for example, the relationships shown below[11,25-28].

$$\ln R = a_0 + a_1 \ln M \tag{1}$$

$$\frac{1}{R} = a_0 + a_1 \frac{1}{M} \tag{2}$$

$$R^2 = a_0 + a_1 M \tag{3}$$

$$R = \frac{R_{max} \cdot M}{K + M} \tag{4}$$

R = relative reflectance
R_{max} = maximum reflectance
M = sample amount
K = constant describing the non-linearity
a_0 and a_1 = constants obtained by linear regression

There are several pitfalls that the analyst should be aware of when using mathematical transformations as it is possible to generate both good and totally erroneous results. These transformations have no theoretical underpinnings and are just another example of curve fitting routines. They tend to work best when the calibration curves are fairly linear to begin with and when the transformation is limited to just a segment of the total calibration curve. Also, it is observed that individual equations may work best for different regions of the same calibration curve and for a series of compounds different equations may have to be used for each curve. There is little singular preference among the proposed equations which must be selected on a substance by substance basis. The linear range of the trans-formed data for estrogen is illustrated in Figure 4. Curve (c) is the extent of the linear range for the raw data (0 to 50ng) while the linear range for equation 1 is 0 to 100ng, equation 2 is 10 to 130ng, and equation 3 is 5 to 150ng. Although good correlation coefficients may be obtained by linear regression it is always necessary to confirm the accuracy of the procedure by back transformation using the new coefficients of the re-gression equation. As the errors are not necessarily transformed equally the transformed calibration curve may be only a poor representation of the original data set.

Calibration in the fluorescence mode rarely causes any problems as calibration curves are usually linear over two to three orders of magni-tude. To preserve the high sample throughput of TLC a novel method of calibration based on the linear relationships found between signal and slit width and the slope of the signal vs. slit width curve and the sample amount in the fluorescence mode has been proposed[29]. The calibration function is described by equation 5.

$$M_u = M_s \frac{S_u}{S_s} \tag{5}$$

M_u = weight of unknown
M_s = weight of standard
S_u = slope of the signal vs. slit width curve for the unknown
S_s = slope of the signal vs. slit width curve for the standard

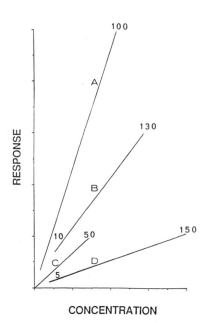

CONCENTRATION

Fig. 4. Linearization of the calibration curve for estrone using (A)
equation (1), (B) equation (2), (C) untransformed data, and (D)
equation (3). Arbitrary units are used for axis.

It was found that S and S could be adequately defined by two values
obtained by scanning each spot with slit widths of 0.4 and 0.8mm. Compared
to normal calibration the accuracy of this method is not as good with
relative errors of 5 to 10% being common. On the other hand, only a single
standard is needed for each substance to be determined, and when multiple
substance calibration is required, all standards can be placed in a single
track leaving the remaining tracks free for samples. This has obvious
advantages for sample screening and the method has been applied to the
quantification of polycyclic aromatic compounds in environmental extracts[30,31].

PHYSICAL AND CHEMICAL METHODS OF FLUORESCENCE ENHANCEMENT TO
IMPROVE SAMPLE DETECTABILITY

     Fluorescence measurements are more selective and sensitive than
absorption and fluorescence calibration curves are generally linear for
reasonable ranges and show much less variation with spot size and shape
than observed with adsorption measurements. However, only a handful of
organic compounds are fluorescent or easily converted into a fluorescent
derivative. For these difficult compounds fluorescence induction is a
convenient alternative. Segura and Gotto noted that heating any involatile
organic substance on a TLC plate at temperatures of 100 to 150°C for 1 to
12h in the presence of ammonium hydrogen carbonate vapors resulted in the
formation of a fluorescent product of consistant fluorescent properties
that were independent of the structure of the treated sample[32]. Apparatus for carrying out fluorescence induction subsequently became commercially available and the method has been applied successfully to the determination of low concentrations of difficult to detect substances such as
drugs, lipids, and amino acids[32-36]. As well as ammonium hydrogen carbonate other Lewis acids or bases such as acid vapors (HCl, HBr, HNO_3,
etc.), silicon tetrachloride, and zirconyl salts have also been used successfully to induce fluorescence[37,38]. As an alternative method to

thermal treatment for fluorescence induction Shanfield et al.[39,40] recommended the use of a gaseous electrical discharge. The discharge treatment produces a higher yield of fluorescent material, is more reproducible and only requires an exposure time of several minutes compared to hours needed by the thermal method. A discharge chamber built in our laboratory is shown in Figure 5. It consists of a glass cylinder with a ground glass joint at the center and has connectors at either end for admitting gases or for evacuating the chamber. The electrical discharge is produced by capacitively coupling a Telsa coil generator to the chamber via a piece of aluminum foil wrapped externally around one part of the tube and a grounded steel wire insulated from the chamber as the counter electrode. We have used this device for a number of years for the qualitative analysis of substances having low UV absorption. The only practical drawback to the technique is that very clean plates and clean working conditions are needed to reduce the general background fluorescence from laboratory contaminants. Also, some plates which incorporate organic binders or containing bonded-layer sorbents cannot be used for obvious reasons.

Along with several other groups we have made several attempts at establishing a mechanism for the fluorescence induction reaction as a first step to optimizing the reaction for quantitative purposes. These have generally fallen on barren ground due to the poor thermal stability of the fluorescent product observed by gas chromatography and its unfavorable chromatographic properties in normal and reversed-phase liquid chromatography. At least this part of the puzzle we have solved recently by using size-exclusion chromatography. In this case peaks of normal shape are observed with an approximate molecular weight of 1,200 to 1,500. Regardless of the composition of the original sample only a single fluorescent product of low polydispersity is formed. However, spectroscopic data provides few real clues to the structure of the polymer which shows little unsaturation, no aromatic groups, and no obvious other functional groups except for possibly hydroxyl groups. Structural elucidation must await further spectroscopic characterization of bulk material which is presently being accumulated using pentanol bonded to silica as substrate and a preparative version of the discharge chamber shown in Figure 5.

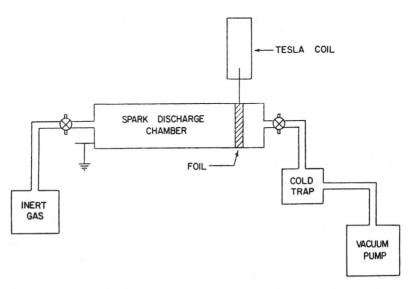

Fig. 5. Discharge chamber for fluorescence induction of organic solutes adsorbed onto silica gel TLC plates.

From time to time a large disparity is observed between the fluorescence properties of a solute in solution and those on a thin-layer plate. These problems usually take the form of fluorescence quenching, shifts in the position of the fluorescence emission, or degradation of the sample to products of low fluorescence efficiency. Impregnating the sample into the sorbent layer provides additional pathways for loss of the excitation energy by non-radiative pathways unavailable in solution. This type of physical interaction can frequently be reversed by dipping or spraying the developed plate with a solution of a viscous liquid such as liquid paraffin[41,42], glycerol[43], cyclodextrin[44], triethanolamine[41], Triton X-100[20,42,45], or Fomblin oil[20,45-47] before detection. The fluorescence enhancement observed is very variable but in favorable cases increases in signal of 10 to 200-fold have been observed. The extent of fluorescent enhancement depends on a number of factors, of which the most important are the sample studied, the characteristics of the sorbent layer, the enhancement reagent used and its concentration, and the time between impregnating the plate with reagent and making measurements. In practice other considerations are equally important such as the extent of spot broadening due to maintaining the sample in a wet layer and shifts in the emission maxima due to changes in the sorbent/sorbate interactions or induced by new interactions between the sorbate and enhancing reagent. Liquids of high viscosity are used as fluorescence enhancing reagents to minimize zone broadening by diffusion and loss in resolution during the time required to scan all samples on the plate.

The importance of chemical reactions for sorbent adsorbed samples is substance dependent. The most common reactions involve catalytic and/or photolytic induced oxidation to products which frequently have a low fluorescence response[46-50]. The rate of fluorescence decay observed under these circumstances is also frequently dependent on the sorbent medium, silica gel plates showing a greater catalytic effect than bonded-phase sorbents in most cases. In several instances incorporating an antioxidant such as BHT (2,6-di-tert-butyl-4-methylphenol) in the mobile phase and using plates impregnated with BHT prior to development will effectively eliminate, or substantially reduce, the decay of the fluorescence signal as a function of time[11]. This is illustrated in Figure 6 for some kinetic data for N,N'-dimethylaminopyrene and aminopyrene. In the absence of BHT the fluorescence signal declines at first rapidly and eventually starts to flatten out. Brief exposure to room fluorescent light after about thirty minutes catalyzes the decay process once again. The sample of N,N'-dimethylaminopyrene protected by BHT shows no variation in response upon prolonged exposure to the atmosphere or upon brief exposure to room lighting.

SOME EMERGING TECHNIQUES FOR QUANTIFICATION AND IDENTIFICATION
IN THIN-LAYER CHROMATOGRAPHY

Current developments in detection methods for TLC are centered around three themes. In situ methods of detection without mechanical scanning using image analyzers, the use of laser sources to enhance sensitivity and selectivity, and hyphenated instruments such as TLC/MS and TLC/FTIR to provide structural information as well as quantification. Compared to slit-scanning densitometry these various methods are at an immature state of development but hold much promise for the future.

Lasers have been used as sources for making fluorescence measurements where their high power and small beam widths could be used to enhance selectivity[51-54]. Selectivity might also be improved by exploring so-called nonlinear fluorescence processes, such as two-photon excited fluorescence and sequentially excited fluorescence, which only become possible

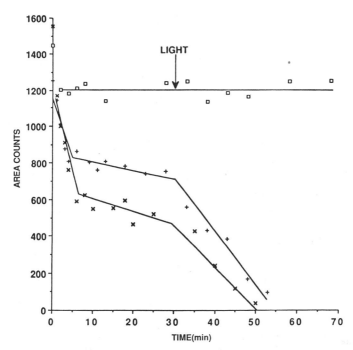

Fig. 6. Photolytic oxidative degradation of N,N'-dimethylaminopyrene in the presence (□), and absence (+) of BHT and aminopyrene (X) on an octadecylsilanized silica TLC plate. The sample was continuously exposed to air but only exposed to room light at the point indicated on the figure.

when laser sources are used. However, to date, laser based densitometers have not demonstrated any significant improvement in sample detectability over densitometers employing conventional arc sources. Since laser beams have small beam widths small imperfections in the sorbent layer make a disproportionate contribution to the noise generated in the measurement. Because of this latter feature most studies have employed lasers operated at only a small fraction of their peak power thus loosing much of the advantage of signal enhancement originally claimed for the laser.

More general success has been achieved using photothermal deflection densitometry, a development arising out of studies on photoacoustic spectroscopy[55-58]. Photothermal deflection spectroscopy involves the measurement of the refractive index gradient formed in the gas phase over a solid sample heated by a laser. If light is absorbed by the sample some of this radiation is converted to heat by radiationless transitions in the sample producing a thermal gradient within the sample and a refractive index change in the layer of air in contact with the sample. This refractive index change is detected by the deflection of a low power laser beam propagating parallel to the plate surface. Detection limits similar to or substantially worse than those obtained by slit-scanning densitometry with conventional sources have been quoted. The actual sensitivity of a particular measurement being a strong function of the method used to detect the signal, the technique used for data transformation, and the wavelength match between the absorption maxima of the sample and the emission line for the heating laser.

The detection process in thin-layer chromatography can be considered static as the sample zones are stationary when the development process is terminated. All information concerning the chromatographic experiment can be made available as a three dimensional array in which the x and y coordinates define the spot position and the z direction the sample amount using image analysis techniques. The equipment requirements for image analysis are a computer with video digitizer, light source and appropriate optics such as lenses, filters, and monochromators, and an imaging detector such as a vidicon tube or charged-coupled video camera[3,59,60]. The plate is evenly illuminated with monochromatic light and the reflected or transmitted light focussed as a scaled image of the plate directly onto the active element of the camera. To obtain wavelength discrimination or to separate excitation and emission wavelengths in the fluorescence mode a monochromator or filters are positioned between the plate and camera. The image resolution is limited by the number of picture elements (pixels), typically 512 x 512 for commercial vidicon cameras, which falls somewhat short of the resolution needed for quantitative two-dimensional TLC. Sensitivity and linearity to response are problems for the simultaneous recording of trace and major components from the same plate.

The future of image analysis as a detection technique for TLC requires the development of both new hardware and software to make it as routine as slit-scanning densitometry. In this respect it is noteworthy that two groups, Read et al., and Kaiser et al., in England and Germany respectively, are already using quantitative image analysis routinely. With technological advances that are occurring quite rapidly in the general area of image analysis, it seems reasonable to anticipate that the current equipment limitations will be solved and in the future commercially produced image analyzers will be available for quantitative TLC at least alongside, or perhaps replacing, slit-scanning densitometers.

One weakness of thin-layer chromatographic methods as practiced today is that they provide insufficient qualitative information to remove any doubt that substances having a specific R_F value could not be incorrectly identified. This is a problem common to all chromatographic techniques that is usually solved by interfacing the chromatographic system to a detector capable of yielding structural information from the sample. Recently some progress has been made in interfacing TLC to infrared spectroscopy, Raman spectroscopy and mass spectrometry in an on-line manner which promises to provide the desirable degree of confidence in substance identification. In general, these techniques are still too insensitive to yield complete spectral features at sample loads typical of modern TLC, but this situation could change presently, as we will see below.

Infrared spectra have been recorded from TLC spots in a alkali halide matrix after either excising the spot before elution or using in situ elution[61]. Spectra are obtained with minimal sample decomposition or contamination in a form suitable for identification from spectral libraries. Typical minimal sample sizes vary from 5 to 50μg for recording full spectral features. A commercial device is available for the in situ recording of infrared spectra of TLC spots by diffuse reflectance FTIR (DRIFT) spectroscopy[63]. For this purpose the spots are positioned manually below the probe beam, diameter 1.0mm, of the attachment. To obtain reasonable spectra the solvent used for development must be scrupulously removed prior to measurement and a correction must be made for the absorption contribution due to the plate. The plate background correction is made by developing two identical plates simultaneously, one plate containing the sample the other acting as the blank. Blank spectra are then subtracted from sample spectra at the same position on both plates. Even with background subtraction one major disadvantage of this technique is that all common TLC media have regions of strong infrared absorption which prevents reliable spectral data being measured in those regions. For silica gel, for example, it is difficult to obtain any useful information in the regions from 3700-3100 and 1650-800cm^{-1}. At least 1µg of material is required to detect individual functional groups and at least ten times this amount for partial spectral recording. Also, compounds bind differently to different sorbents and this is usually reflected in changes in band positions which makes spectral interpretation less reliable without reference spectra obtained on the same sorbent.

Infrared spectra have also been recorded using photoaucoustic spectroscopy (PAS). PAS spectra are usually measured by enclosing the sample in a fixed volume cell. The sample is then illuminated through a window with chopped monochromatic radiation. The radiant energy absorbed by the sample is converted to heat which flows to the surrounding gas and generates a pressure pulse that is detected with a microphone connected to the sample chamber. The output from the microphone is fed to a lock-in-amplifier referenced at the frequency of the source radiation. The PAS absorption spectra is then generated by plotting the lock-in-amplifier signal as a function of the wavelength of the incident radiation. The PAS method, however, suffers from all the same problems as discussed for DRIFT spectra; namely strong interference and/or absorption by solvent vapors and the sorbent medium[64,65].

Surface enhanced Raman spectroscopy (SERS) is unaffected by the problems due to moisture and background absorption that plague infrared techniques[66,67]. The sensitivity and spatial resolving power of the technique are compatible with the modern practice of TLC. Reasonable spectra can be obtained from as little as 10 to 60ng of sample per spot. Compared to solution spectra changes in band intensities and position are sometimes observed for the sorbent adsorbed species. Further work is required to define the optimum parameters for recording spectra, for example, whether a postchromatographic treatment with a silver colloid is needed as claimed in one report[67]. Notwithstanding these procedural difficulties, the method holds a great deal of promise for the future.

Several methods have been used to obtain mass spectra from TLC spots. Excising sample spots and direct insertion of sample plus sorbent into the ion source of the mass spectrometer generally requires relatively high temperatures for desorption and large sample amounts to give a usable mass spectra. Polar and high molecular weight samples are not easily desorbed and elution of the sample from the sorbent prior to insertion into the ion source is generally preferred for these samples. Fast atom bombardment (FAB) mass spectra of thermally labile and involatile samples can be obtained directly from TLC plates[68]. The standard FAB probe is covered with a strip of double-sided masking tape and the tip of the probe pressed against the TLC spot to lift it from the plate. Small volumes of solvent and FAB matrix solution, a few µL, are then added to the sorbent and the probe inserted into the ion chamber in the usual way.

A direct interface for obtaining chemical ionization mass spectra from spots on various types of TLC plates has also been described[69,70]. A scanning device is used to move the TLC plate past a source of desorption energy, either a low power pulsed carbon dioxide laser or tungsten filament incandescent lamp. The chemical ionization gas is then used to sweep the desorbed materials through a heated inlet system into the ion source of a quadrupole mass spectrometer. The laser method provides very little bulk heating of the plate and is preferred to the incandescent filament when compounds of limited thermal stability and low volatility are to be examined. From studies of model compounds it was shown that polar and high molecular weight compounds are only poorly transferred to the mass spectrometer. This may be due to inefficient desorption from the plate or recondensation on cold spots within the scanner unit. Compounds with molecular weights greater than 200 showed a considerable decrease in sensitivity compared to lower molecular weight compounds and few compounds with molecular weights greater than 300 could be detected at all. In favorable cases detection limits of about 1.0ng were obtained by single ion monitoring and about 10ng when a small mass range was scanned. However, the precision was very poor when attempts were made to make quantitative measurements of TLC spots.

Recently, it has been shown that surface ionization techniques can be used to obtain characteristic mass spectra from the few atom layers of sample associated with the sorbent surface[71,72]. The mass spectra obtained by surface ionization mass spectrometry (SIMS) typically contain even-electron ions of the same type observed in chemical ionization mass spectra and the fragmentation processes observed are analogous in many cases. In the SIMS experiment the scrupulously dry plate in a vacuum chamber is scanned through an ion beam using a motor driven scanning stage similar in principle to scanning densitometry. The primary ion beam, usually argon or cesium, is accelerated to high energy and collides with the surface transferring its energy in a collision cascade to atoms and molecules in the surface region. Neutral molecules, ions, electrons, and photons are ejected from the surface. The ions of interest are drawn into the mass spectrometer by an extraction potential where they are analyzed. The sensitivity of the technique can be improved by using a phase transition matrix and time averaging[73]. Since ions are removed only from the surface the bulk of the sample is not ionized by the primary ion beam unless a mechanism can be found to extract and cycle the major portion of the sample to the surface in a continuous manner. Impregnating the chromatogram with a viscous liquid or low melting point solid such as glycerol or 1,2,3,4-butanetetrol extracts the sample from the sorbent and allows its vertical movement to the surface where ionization occurs (the primary ion beam provides sufficient energy to melt the solid matrix in the neighborhood of its point of impact. This provides extraction without zone broadening). By using a phase transition matrix a steady signal can be obtained for several hours permitting extended data collection and lowering of the sensitivity of the technique to the tens of nanogram range. More usual sample sizes for obtaining a full mass spectra without averaging are in the microgram range.

CONCLUSIONS

It is the authors' opinion that for the present time slit-scanning densitometry will remain the primary quantitative technique in TLC. Sufficient information is known concerning the general parameters of the technique that its routine use, with regard to this framework, should present few problems. Electronic scanning, using image analyzers, clearly offers many potential benefits, but with todays technology base, their performance is not competitive with conventional slit-scanning densitometers. Their time may come, however, and only a comparatively moderate enhancement in technology is needed to make their use practical and competitive to conventional densitometers. It is less clear what advances can be anticipated from in situ infrared methods but Raman (SERS) and mass spectrometry (SIMS) should make hyphenated methods incorporating modern TLC practical in the near future.

REFERENCES

1. C. F. Poole, Trends Anal.Chem. 4:209 (1985).
2. C. F. Poole, S. Khatib, and T. A. Dean, Chromatogr.Forum 1:27 (1986).
3. C. F. Poole and S. K. Poole, in: "Multidimensional Chromatography:

Techniques and Applications", H. J. Cortes ed., Marcel Dekker, New York, in press, (1988).

4. C. F. Poole and S. A. Schuette, "Contemporary Practice of Chromatography," p. 619, Elsevier, Amsterdam (1984).

5. R. E. Kaiser, (ed.), "Planar Chromatography," vol. 1, Heuthig, Heidelberg (1986).

6. W. Bertsch, S. Hara, R. E. Kaiser, and A. Zlatkis, (eds.), "Instrumental HPTLC," Huethig, Heidelberg (1980).

7. M. E. Coddens, H. T. Butler, S. A. Schuette, and C. F. Poole, LC-GC Magzn. 1:282 (1983).

8. C. F. Poole, H. T. Butler, M. E. Coddens, and S. A. Schuette, in: "Analytical And Chromatographic Techniques in Radiopharamaceutical Chemistry," p. 3, D. M. Wieland, T. J. Manger, and M. C. Tobes, eds., Springer-Verlag, New York, (1985).

9. I. M. Bohrer, Topics Current Chem., 126:95 (1984).

10. V. Pollak, Adv.Chromatogr., 17:1 (1979).

11. C. F. Poole and S. Khatib, in: "Quantitative Analysis Using Chromatographic Techniques," p. 193, E. D. Katz, ed., John Wiley, Chichester (1987).

12. S. Ebel and E. Glaser, J.High Resolut.Chromatogr.Chromatogr.Commun., 2:36 (1979).

13. S. J. Costanzo and M. J. Cardone, J.Liquid Chromatogr., 7:2711 (1984).

14. D. C. Fenimore, in: "Instrumental HPTLC," W. Bertsch, S. Hara, R. E. Kaiser, and A. Zlatkis, eds., p. 81 Huethig, Heidelberg, (1980).

15. D. C. Fenimore and C. J. Meyer, J.Chromatogr., 186:555 (1979).

16. A. Karmen, G. Malikin, L. Freundlich, and S. Lam, J.Chromatogr., 349:267 (1985).

17. H. Bethke, W. Santi, and R. W. Frei, J.Chromatogr.Sci., 12:392 (1974).

18. H. Yamamoto, T. Kurita, J. Suzuki, R. Hira, and K. Shibata, J.Chromatogr. 116:29 (1976).

19. H. T. Butler, S. A. Schuette, F. Pacholec, and C. F. Poole, J.Chromatogr., 261:55 (1983).

20. C. F. Poole, M. E. Coddens, H. T. Butler, S. A. Schuette, S. S. J. Ho, S. Khatib, L. Piet, and K. K. Brown, J.Liq.Chromatogr., 8:2875 (1985).

21. M. E. Coddens, S. Khatib, H. T. Butler, and C. F. Poole, J.Chromatogr., 280:15 (1983).

22. H. T. Butler and C. F. Poole, J.High Resolut.Chromatogr.Chromatogr., Commun., 6:77 (1983).

23. M. E. Coddens and C. F. Poole, Anal.Chem., 55:2429 (1983).

24. M. E. Coddens and C. F. Poole, LC-GC Magzn. 2:34 (1984).

25. S. Ebel, Topics Current Chem., 126:71 (1984).

26. S. Ebel, D. Alert, and U. Schaefer, Chromatographia, 18:23 (1984).

27. N. Sistovaris, Trends Anal.Chem., 5:158 (1986).

28. S. Khatib and C. F. Poole, LC-GC Magzn., 4:228 (1983).

29. H. T. Butler and C. F. Poole, J.Chromatogr.Sci., 21:385 (1983).

30. H. T. Butler, M. E. Coddens, S. Khatib, and C. F. Poole, J.Chromatogr. Sci., 23:200 (1985).

31. S. K. Poole, T. A. Dean, and C. F. Poole, J.Chromatogr., 400:323 (1987).

32. R. Segura and A. M. Gotto, J.Chromatogr., 99:643 (1974).

33. T. Hagiwara, S. Higeoka, S. Uehara, N. Miyatake, and K. Akiyama, J.High Resolut.Chromatogr.Chromatogr.Commun., 7:161 (1984).

34. E.-M. Karlson and H. W. Peter, J.Chromatogr., 155:218 (1978).

35. I. R. Kupke and S. Zeugner, J.Chromatogr., 146:261 (1978).

36. L. Zhou, H. Shanfield and A. Zlatkis, J.Chromatogr. 239:258 (1982).

37. L. Zhou, H. Shanfield, F.-S. Wang, and A. Zlatkis, J.Chromatogr., 217:341 (1981).

38. R. Segura and X. Navarro, J.Chromatogr., 217:329 (1981).

39. H. Shanfield, F. Hsu, and A. J. P. Martin, J.Chromatogr., 126:457 (1976).

40. H. Shanfield, K. Y. Lee, and A. J. P. Martin, J.Chromatogr., 142:387 (1977).
41. W. Funk, R. Kerler, J. Th. Schiller, V. Dammann, and F. Arndt, J.High Resolut.Chromatogr.Chromatogr.Commun., 5:534 (1982).
42. D. Woolbeck, E. V. Kleist, I. E. Elmadfa, and W. Funk, J.High Resolut.Chromatogr.Chromatogr.Commun., 7:473 (1984).
43. S. Uchiyama and M. Uchiyama, J.Chromatogr., 262:240 (1980).
44. A. Alak, E. Heilweil, W. L. Hinze, H. Oh, and D. W. Armstrong, J.Liquid Chromatogr., 7:1273 (1984).
45. S. S. J. Ho, H. T. Butler, and C. F. Poole, J.Chromatogr., 281:330 (1983).
46. K. K. Brown and C. F. Poole, LC-GC Magzn., 2:526 (1984).
47. K. K. Brown and C. F. Poole, J.High Resolut,Chromatogr.Chromatogr., Commun., 7:520 (1984).
48. B. Seifert, J.Chromatogr., 131:417 (1977).
49. H. Fabre, M.-D. Blanchin, D. Lerner, and B. Mandrau, Analyst 110:775 (1985).
50. J. N. Miller, Pure & Appl.Chem., 57:515 (1985).
51. M. K. L. Bicking, R. N. Kniseley, and J. J. Svec, Anal.Chem., 55:200 (1983).
52. P. B. Huffand and M. J. Sepaniak, Anal.Chem., 55:1994 (1983).
53. M. L. K. Bicking, in: "Techniques and Applications of Thin-Layer Chromatography," p. 1, J. C. Touchstone and J. Sherma, eds., Wiley, New York (1985).
54. B. G. Belenki, E. S. Gankina, T. B. Adamovich, A. Ph. Lobazov, S. V. Nechaev, and M. G. Solonenko, J.Chromatogr., 365:315 (1986).
55. F. K. Fortiou and M. D. Morris, Anal.Chem., 59:185 (1987).
56. K. Peck, F. K. Fotiou, and M. D. Morris, Anal.Chem., 57:1359 (1985).
57. T. I. Chen and M. D. Morris, Anal.Chem., 56:19 (1984).
58. T. Masujima, A. N. Sharda, L. B. Lloyd, J. M. Harris, and E. M. Eyring, Anal.Chem., 56:2975 (1984).
59. D. H. Burns, J. B. Callis, and G. D. Christian, Trends Anal.Chem., 5:50 (1986).
60. S. Pongor, J.Liq.Chromatogr., 5:1583 (1982).
61. K. H. Shafer, P. R. Griffiths, and W. Shu-Qin, Anal.Chem., 58:2708 (1986).
62. J. M. Chalmers, M. W. Mackenzie, J. L. Sharp, and R. N. Ibbett, Anal.Chem., 59:415 (1987).
63. G. E. Zuber, R. J. Warren, P. P. Begash, and E. L. O'Donnel Anal.Chem., 56:2935 (1984).
64. R. L. White, Anal.Chem., 57:1819 (1985).
65. L. B. Lloyd, R. C. Yeates, and E. M. Eyring, Anal.Chem., 54:549 (1982).
66. D. W. Armstrong, L. A. Spino, M. R. Ondrias, and E. W. Findsen, J.Chromatogr., 369:227 (1986).
67. J.-M. L. Sequaris and E. Koglin. Anal.Chem., 59:525 (1987).
68. T. T. Chang, J. O. Lay, and R. J. Francel, Anal.Chem., 56:109 (1984).
69. L. Ramaley, M. E. Nearing, M.-A. Vaughn, R. G. Ackman, and W. D. Jamisen, Anal.Chem., 55:2285 (1983).
70. L. Ramaley, M.-A. Vaughn, and W. D. Jamieson, Anal.Chem., 57:353 (1985).
71. J. W. Fiola, G. C. DiDonato, and K. L. Busch. Rev.Scient.Instrum., 57:2294 (1986).
72. K. L. Busch. Trends Anal.Chem., 6:95 (1987).
73. G. C. DiDonato and K. L. Busch, Anal.Chem., 58:3231 (1986).

FLUORESCENCE LINE-NARROWING SPECTROSCOPY: A NEW AND
HIGHLY SELECTIVE DETECTION TECHNIQUE FOR THIN-LAYER
AND LIQUID CHROMATOGRAPHY

J. W. Hofstraat, C. Gooijer, U. A. Th. Brinkman
and N. H. Velthorst

Department of General and Analytical Chemsitry
Free University, De Boelelaan 1083, 1081, HV Amsterdam
The Netherlands

SUMMARY

Fluorescence line-narrowing spectroscopy, a technique that makes use
of laser excitation of molecules in low temperature solid matrices to
obtain vibrationally resolved fluorescence spectra, can be successfully
applied for the analysis of compounds on thin-layer chromatographic (TLC)
plates. Consequently this technique is suitable as a highly specific
detection method in TLC. It is also shown that TLC plates can be used as
buffer-memory for column liquid chromatography (LC). The stored chromatogram can be cooled and subsequently probed with the laser beam. In this
way fluorescence line-narrowing can also be employed as off-line detection
method in LC.

INTRODUCTION

Fluorescence spectroscopy is a widely applied detection technique in
both thin-layer chromatography (TLC) and column liquid chromatography (LC).
It is especially useful for the quantitative determination of molecules at
trace levels, because of its high sensitivity. However, for qualitative
analysis fluorescence spectroscopy is much less useful.

The electronic emission (and absorption) spectra of molecules in
liquid solutions in general are broad and featureless and thus not very
selective. Spectral bandwidths can be 10 to 50nm, so that the vibronic
fine structure of the fluorescence spectrum is hardly discernible. These
bandwidths are very much larger than the minimum bandwidth physically
achievable, the so-called natural bandwidth which is only determined by the
lifetimes of the states involved in the transition according to the
Heisenberg uncertainty relation[1]. For fluorescence transitions the
lifetime of the excited state generally lies in the low nanosecond range,
while the ground state has infinite lifetime, so that the limiting bandwidth is in the order of 10^{-5}nm. The broadening of the spectral bands in
liquid solutions is mainly caused by rapidly changing, varying interactions
of the dissolved molecules with the solvent molecules surrounding them,
that lead to shifts in the solute energy levels. At present no techniques
are available to substantially reduce the broadening of fluid state fluorescence spectra. The changes in solvent structure occur on a much faster

time scale than the lifetime of the excited state so that there seems to be no way to reduce the bandwidth in this case.

Even for frozen solutions, generally broad-banded spectra are obtained, though all major movements of the solvent molecules on the fluorescence time scale have stopped (cf. the spectrum of pyrene shown in Figure 1a). This has to be ascribed to the heterogeneous structure of most solid solutions. The inhomogeneous broadening of low temperature solid state spectra, however, can be reduced by bringing a well defined distribution of molecules to the excited state via laser excitation[1,2]: only those molecules that have an energy difference between ground and excited state that coincides with the laser photon energy are excited, and only those molecules will be able to fluoresce. If the excited state energy distribution remains pure until emission takes place, this fluorescence signal will be narrow banded so that vibrational resolution is obtained. For this fluorescence line-narrowing (FLN) spectroscopy technique two conditions have to be fulfilled:

1. The temperature of the solution must be below 30-50 K to prevent spectral diffusion processes and to reduce the influence of the coupling of the solute electronic transition with the collective vibrations of the matrix molecules (phonons). Electron-phonon coupling leads to the appearance of broad bands next to the narrow lines in the FLN spectrum. At lower temperatures less of the low energy phonon states are populated so that these broad bands are less intense.

2. Excitation should take place into the S_1-S_0 0-0 transition (i.e. in a crude approximation: the electronic state changes, but the vibrational state does not) or into low-energy vibronically excited S_1 states (less than about $1500cm^{-1}$ above the 0-0 transition). Probing the higher energy vibronic region, where the density of states is large, complicated spectra arise as many distributions of excited molecules are created via excitation in numerous vibronic states. Excitation into higher excited states (S_2, etc.) leads to broad-banded spectra, as these states have extremely short lifetimes and thus very large natural bandwidths.

If the conditions mentioned above are fulfilled, vibrationally resolved spectra can be obtained, which have the same high specificity as infrared spectra and the high sensitivity that is typical for fluorescence spectra.

In this paper we will discuss the application of the FLN technique as detection method in TLC and as off-line detection method in LC. FLN spectroscopy is not suitable for on-line detection in LC, since its requirement of a solid matrix is obviously not compatible with a flowing, dynamic system. To overcome this problem resort was made to immobilization of the effluent of the LC system on a TLC plate. The stored chromatograms can subsequently be cooled and investigated with the FLN technique.

EXPERIMENTAL

FLN spectra were recorded at about 10K in a Cryodyne model 21 closed cycle helium refrigerator of CTI Cryogenics (Waltham, MA, USA). A Coherent (Palo Alto, CA, USA) CR 10 argon-ion laser was used for excitation; for the pyrenes the 363.8nm laser line was used, for tetracene the 457.9nm line. Detection was performed with a Jarrell-Ash (Waltham, MA, USA) 82-000 0.5 m monochromator and a Princeton Applied Research (Princeton, NJ, USA) HR-8 lock-in amplifier or with a Jeol (Tokyo, Japan) JRS 400D double monochromator followed by a Jeol photon counting system. Typical instrumental bandwidths used were 0.05-0.1 nm.

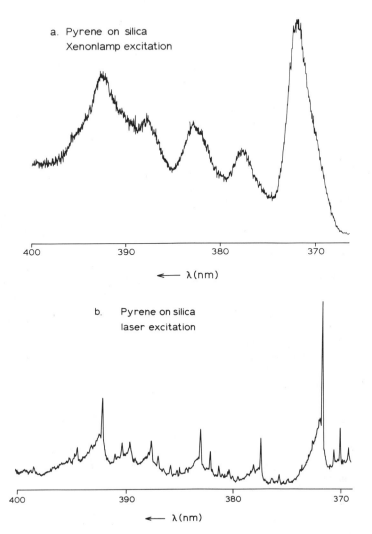

Fig. 1. (a) Fluorescence spectrum of 7µg of pyrene on a silica TLC plate
with broad-band lamp excitation at 320 nm (T = 20 K). (b) FLN
spectrum of 0.6 µg of pyrene on a silica TLC plate with laser
excitation at 363.8 nm (T = 20 K).

As model compounds tetracene, pyrene and 1-fluoropyrene were chosen.
Matrix materials were precoated silica and C_{18}-modified silica TLC plates
from Merck (Darmstadt, FRG). Solutions of the model compounds were either
applied with a microliter syringe or with the LC/TLC interface. As interface a modified CAMAG (Muttenz, Switzerland) Linomat III line applicator
for TLC was used. The eluent from a narrow-bore LC column was led through
a fused silica capillary that protruded from the spray jet assembly of the
Linomat. The eluent jet was sprayed on a TLC plate placed on a moveable
table. Both normal-phase and reversed-phase LC was applied; n-hexane and
methanol/water (9:1, v/v) were used as eluents. Flow rates varied between
10 and 40 µl/min.

RESULTS AND DISCUSSION

Application of FLN as Detection Method in TLC

Recently it has been shown that FLN spectra can be obtained for compounds on TLC plates cooled to cryogenic temperatures[4-5]. As an example
the spectrum of pyrene on a silica TLC plate (laser excitation 363.8nm) is
represented in Figure 1b. The impressive improvement in resolution as
compared to the spectrum depicted in Figure 1a, where a conventional xenon
lamp is used for excitation, is clear. The FLN spectrum exhibits a wealth
of narrow lines that reflect the vibrational structure of the ground state
of the molecule. The three bands at the high energy side are 0-0 transitions. As excitation is performed into the vibronic S_1 region the laser
photons will produce several distributions of excited molecules, since they
will coincide with a number of inhomogeneously broadened vibrationally
excited S_1 bands that will all relax to their corresponding vibrational
ground states.

The high selectivity of the FLN method is clearly visible in Figure 2,
where the 0-0 region of the fluorescence spectrum of a mixture of pyrene
and 1-fluoropyrene is depicted. The transitions of the two strongly related compounds can be distinguished very well: the main band of pyrene is
found at 371.8nm, 1-fluoropyrene shows two strong bands at 372.0 and
374.2nm. Even though the transitions of these molecules are separated by
only 0.2nm they can be readily identified. The width of the spectral bands
in FLN spectra in general is below 0.1nm; it is largely determined by the
instrumental bandwidth employed (the laser bandwidth is generally below
0.01nm). Furthermore the reproducibility of the spectral wavelength positions is very good, as it is mainly determined by the wavelength reproducibility of the laser.

Due to the complexity of our present experimental set-up, reproducible
optical alignment is very difficult, so that for quantification purposes an
internal standard had to be added. This method provides satisfactory
calibration curves, as shown in Figure 2. In this plot the intensity of
the 374.2nm band of 1-fluoropyrene, deposited in different amounts, is
weighted with the 371.8nm band of pyrene. The correlation coefficient is

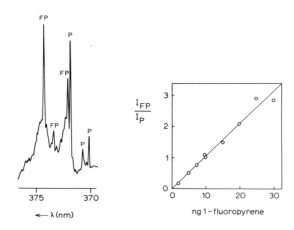

Fig. 2. FLN spectrum of the 0-0 transition area of a mixture of 25 ng of
         1-fluoropyrene (FP) and 40 ng of pyrene (P) on a silica TLC plate
         with laser excitation at 363.8 nm at T = 20 K (left). Calibration
         curve for 1-fluoropyrene in the low concentration region (right);
         explanation, see text.

0.99 (n=10). The reproducibility of each determination, measured for five, separately applied, identical sample spots was better than 8%. The analytical curve is linear from the detection limit, which is approximately 1ng, to about 100ng, i.e. over two orders of magnitude. At higher concentrations excimer fluorescence is observed for pyrene, producing a broad band around 470nm and reabsorption of the narrow 0-0 lines occurs. Although the total amount of pyrene on the TLC plate is not large, the effective concentration can be quite high due to the small amount of TLC material that is occupied (the average spot has a diameter of about 1mm).

The detection limit is mainly determined by the laser stray light that obscures the weak fluorescence signals. In Figure 1b the effect of stray light is visible in the slightly increasing intensity of the baseline at shorter wavelengths. However, the detection limit can be improved considerably. Experiments with tetracene on TLC plates, in which a double monochromator was used which has excellent stray light rejection properties, have revealed detection limits in the low picogram range[6]. Further improvements can be obtained by employing a tunable dye laser (so that the excitation wavelength can be tuned to an intense absorption band), by making use of spraying techniques, or by using other TLC materials to enhance the fluorescence signal. It has been shown that spraying a silica TLC plate with an n-alkane, or the use of alkyl-modified TLC materials, can increase the intensity of the bands in the FLN spectrum by as much as one order of magnitude. Under optimal circumstances detection limits in the femtogram range may therefore be attainable.

Application of FLN as detection method following a TLC separation has been demonstrated for a mixture of chloropyrenes[5]. FLN spectra were obtained after elution with cyclohexane/hexane (1:1, v/v) on a silica TLC plate for the separated compounds. However, as a consequence of the high specificity of the method it appeared also possible to identify the compounds without separation. For complicated samples, with increasing spectral interferences, a combination of TLC separation and FLN detection will be more useful.

Application of FLN as Detection Method in LC

A direct application of FLN as detection technique in LC is obviously impossible: a way has to be found to store the separated compounds so that cooling and probing with the laser is feasible. The use of TLC plates as buffer-memory for LC was prompted by the observation, illustrated above, that good FLN spectra can be obtained for molecules in such media. The coupling of LC and TLC, however, can also serve other means. After deposition of the compounds separated in LC on a TLC plate the chromatogram remains conserved. Thus it is available for another separation step and/or for further study. For instance, detection methods that cannot be applied in LC because they are rather slow (like infrared spectroscopy or fluorescence and absorption scanning methods) or incompatible with fluid systems (like phosphorescence, surface-enhanced Raman spectroscopy or low-temperature solid-state techniques as FLN spectroscopy) can now readily be applied. The scope of the LC-TLC coupling therefore goes far beyond the application discussed here.

As the way in which the LC effluent is deposited on the TLC plate is crucial for the extent to which the chromatographic information of the initial separation is conserved, this interface has been thoroughly evaluated[3]. It appears that the effluent from a narrow-bore LC column can be deposited on a TLC plate after a normal-phase as well as a reversed-phase separation without serious loss of chromatographic resolution. Both silica and alkyl-modified silica TLC plates can be used for storage. The deposition of the analytes on the TLC material is strongly influenced by their R_F values for the particular combination of TLC material and eluent, the migration behaviour of the eluent on the TLC material and the volatility of the eluent. The best results obviously are obtained for highly volatile eluents with minimal migration on the TLC material. All these factors are to a great extent determined by external circumstances, like the type of compounds that have to be separated, which will, for instance, fix the choice of LC separation. The storage process can also be influenced by a number of factors that can be chosen by the chemist. These are:

1. Varying the amount of effluent stored per unit of surface area of the TLC plate, which can be done through the LC flow rate and the speed of the Linomat table. An optimum has to be found here as small amounts per mm^2 are favourable for storage but unfavourable for sensitivity.
2. Varying the distance of the outlet of the jet to the TLC plate.
3. Varying the nitrogen gas flow which is fed to the jet to improve the evaporation of the eluent; apart from changing the gas pressure also heating of the gas can be applied.
4. Heating of the column effluent or the TLC plate.

In Figure 3 an example is shown of the results which are obtained for the deposition of the effluent from a normal-phase LC separation (eluent n-hexane) at a flow rate of $30\mu l/min$ on a silica TLC plate moving with a speed of 13.7 mm/min. The chromatogram that was obtained with a UV absorption detector (250nm) placed in the LC system directly after the separation column is shown in Figure 3a whilst Figure 3b shows the corresponding TLC-stored chromatogram. This clearly illustrates that the chromatographic resolution remains well conserved after deposition. The retention times of the compounds measured on the TLC plate are about 30 sec longer than measured in the LC experiment, which corresponds with a dead volume of about $15\mu l$ after the UV absorption detector. Most of the increase in bandwidth observed after deposition (about 40-50 sec^2 width at half maximum for the model compounds used) can be attributed to this dead volume. Recent experiments have shown that by a careful optimization of the deposition circumstances, storage on the TLC plate can be realized without any increase in bandwidth[7]

The spectrum shown in Figure 4 represents that which is obtained for the model compound tetracene which was deposited on a silica TLC plate in the experiment shown in Figure 3. Clearly application of FLN as off-line detection method for LC becomes feasible when TLC plates are employed for storage. The same considerations as mentioned in the previous section for the use of FLN as detection method in TLC hold for this case, only the mode of application of the compounds on the TLC plate differs.

CONCLUSIONS

FLN spectroscopy can be used as detection method for compounds on TLC plates. This technique provides highly specific, vibrationally resolved spectra at sensitivities approximating those of conventional fluorescence spectroscopy. Detection limits in the high femtogram to low picogram range are estimated for molecules with high fluorescence quantum yields under optimal experimental circumstances.

The FLN technique can also be used for detection in micro-LC. It appears possible to immobilize compounds separated in a micro-LC column on a TLC plate without serious loss of chromatographic resolution. The storage process can be successfully applied in a combination with normal-phase and reversed-phase separations, even if the eluent in the latter case contains water.

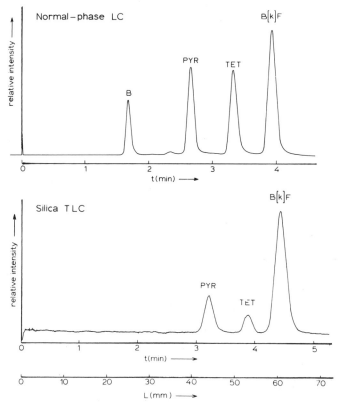

Fig. 3. Normal-phase LC coupled to silica TLC for a mixture containing
benzene (B), 5.7 ng of pyrene (PYR), 13 ng of tetracene (TET) and
3.5 ng of benz[k]fluoranthene (B[k]F). The LC flow-rate was 30
μl/min, the Linomat table speed 13.7 mm/min. (a) On-line liquid
chromatogram with UV (250 nm) absorption detection. (b) Stored
liquid chromatogram with fluorescence detection.

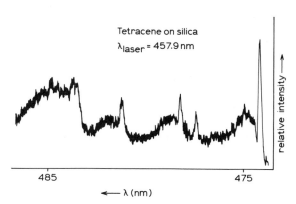

Fig. 4. FLN spectrum of 13 ng of tetracene after storage on a silica TLC
plate. Laser excitation at 457.9 nm was applied. Temperature was
10 K.

REFERENCES

1. J. W. Hofstraat, C. Gooijer and N. H. Velthorst, in: "Methods in Molecular Spectroscopy," S. G. Schulman ed., vol. 2, Wiley, New York, to appear in 1987.

2. R. I. Personov, in: "Spectroscopy and Excitation Dynamics of Condensed Molecular Systems," V. M. Agranovich and R. M. Hochstrasser, eds., North-Holland, ch. 10, p. 555, Amsterdam (1983).

3. J. W. Hofstraat, M. Engelsma, R. J. van de Nesse, C. Gooijer, N. H. Velthorst and U. A. Th. Brinkman, Anal.Chim.Acta., 186:247 (1986).

4. J. W. Hofstraat, M. Engelsma, W. P. Cofino, G.Ph. Hoornweg, C. Gooijer and N. H. Velthorst, Anal.Chim.Acta., 159:359 (1984).

5. J. W. Hofstraat, H. J. M. Jansen, G.Ph. Hoornweg, C. Gooijer and N.H. Velthorst, Anal.Chim.Acta., 170:61 (1985).

6. J. W. Hofstraat, M. Engelsma, R. J. van de Nesse, U. A. Th. Brinkman, C. Gooijer and N. H. Velthorst, Anal.Chim.Acta., 193:193 (1987).

7. J. W. Hofstraat, J. W. Griffioen, U. A. Th. Brinkman, C. Gooijer and N. H. Velthorst, in preparation.

QUALITATIVE AND QUANTITATIVE IMAGE ANALYSIS OF FLUORESCENCE

FROM HIGH PERFORMANCE THIN-LAYER CHROMATOGRAPHY

R. M. Belchamber, S. J. Brinkworth
H. Read and J. D. M. Roberts

BP Research Centre
Sunbury-on-Thames, Middlesex TW16 7LN, UK

SUMMARY

A solid state video camera and an image processing system consisting
of a frame store and computer have been used to analyze images of HPTLC
plates. The images can be obtained using transmission or reflectantance
mode illumination. Some spectral selectivity can be introduced by using
appropriate Wratten type filters. Fluorescent compounds can be imaged by
UV illumination.

The images were enhanced using digital filtering techniques, contrast
stretching, image ratioing, averaging and false color. This enhancement
enables "finger-print" comparisons of complex mixtures to be easily made.

Images were then corrected for variation in illumination intensity.
The data was then treated by a chain contouring algorithm, which was used
to detect spots, followed by the automatic determination of their luminance
intensity. The intensity of the spot could then be directly related to the
concentration of the components of interest. Using this technique quantitative determinations have been obtained for components in complex samples.

INTRODUCTION

With the advent of new stationary phases, chromatographic development
methods and microprocessor instrumentation, high performance thin-layer
chromatography (HPTLC) has become a widespread laboratory technique. This
has enabled the analyst to separate complex samples cost effectively and
quickly. However, a major limiting factor has been the relatively long
time required to perform quantitative analysis. Conventional scanning
densitometers may be used to scan along a preset linear or zig-zag path on
linearly and radially eluted plates. When scanning in the zig-zag mode,
which is necessary for radial plates and plates with poorly defined spots,
very long scanning times may be required. The speed of densitometry poses
a problem when the visualized components are unstable. For instance, when
working with compounds that have been labelled by forming fluorescent
adducts, a scan of the entire plate is not always possible as the time
required can be greater than the lifetime of the fluorescent species.

A number of papers have been published describing a variety of video camera systems for the analysis of planar chromatography plates[1-19]. We have previously used such a system for the qualitative and quantitative analysis of HPTLC plates in the visible region[1,2]. This system consisted of a modified charge coupled device camera and an image processing system. This method has the advantage that plate scanning is essentially instantaneous and the data produced is in a form highly suited to mathematical manipulation. This allows the images to be enhanced for visual assessment and provides the ability to automatically extract quantitative information.

In this paper an image integration or averaging technique to acquire high contrast quantitative images of weakly fluorescing compounds separated by HPTLC is described.

EXPERIMENTAL

Samples and Reagents

Detergent samples (aryl sulphonates) blended in an oil matrix were obtained from commercial suppliers. All solvents used were redistilled analytical grade. Photoquality pinacryptol yellow (Fluka) was used to form fluorescent adducts.

Chromatographic Method

The HPTLC was carried out on silica gel F254 plates impregnated with an inorganic fluorescent agent. Samples were applied using a Linomat IV (Camag) sample applicator and developed in the HPTLC linear development chamber (Camag). Plates were eluted (50mm) with a toluene: methanol mixture (80:20 v/v). The aryl sulphonates were labelled by forming a fluorescent pinacryptol yellow ion-pair adduct. This was achieved by dipping the plate, after elution, in a solution of pinacryptol yellow in ethanol (1% w/v).

Image Acquisition and Processing

The image processing system consisted of a solid state video camera (charge-coupled device, Pulnix TM-46), a 512 x 512 pixels x 8 bit framestore (Intellect 100, Quantel Ltd, Newbury, Berkshire, UK), a minicomputer (PDP 11/23, Digital Equipment Corporation) and a high resolution color monitor. After capture and processing, images were stored for further processing and future reference as 'bit maps' on a 10.5 M-byte disc (RL-02, Digital Equipment Corporation). This system has previously been described in detail[2].

The plates were illuminated by a single UV lamp (365 nm). The camera lens, the plate and the light source were contained in a dark box.

Software for image acquisition and processing was written in FORTRAN IV and made use of the library routines supplied with the framestore.

The following sequence of operations was performed to acquire, enhance and analyze the image of the plate.

1. A freshly developed plate was dipped in the pinacryptol yellow solution, dried and positioned under the camera.

2. A recursive image processing routine was then invoked which integrated successive frames to build up a high quality image in the framestore memory. The framestore was set into '16 bit mode', which means that two

8 bit memory locations were used to contain one 16 bit word. Only odd numbered pixels, which correspond to the high order byte of this word are
displayed. Live 8 bit images were then added successively to the even
pixels. Only as the accumulated total spills over into the higher 8 bits,
i.e. the odd pixels, does it appear on the monitor. To obtain images from
weakly fluorescing components typically 800 images would be integrated in
this manner. This takes 33 seconds using the present equipment. After
integration the odd pixels are duplicated into their adjacent even numbered
counterparts, which are then also displayed. The background luminance
level is subtracted from each pixel and the image is rescaled to fill the 8
bit dynamic range of the framestore.

3.   Quantitative determinations were made either by directly measuring the
maximum intensities of the spots or using a chain contouring algorithm
which defines the spot boundaries and sums the intensity values of the
enclosed pixels[2]. Other processing techniques such as digital filtering
and pseudo-color representations can be used to further improve the quality
of the image presentation[1,2].

RESULTS

A single video image obtained of a plate used to separate an aryl
sulphonate from a hydrocarbon base oil is shown in Figure 1. Averaging 800
of these images produced an image which exhibited a much higher contrast
and better signal-to-noise ratio characteristics, as shown in Figure 2.
The sulphonate was present at various concentrations (0.03, 0.15, 0.23,
0.3, 0.45, and 0.6% w/v). A calibration curve was obtained by plotting the
maximum intensity of each spot against concentration (Figure 3). A good
quantitative relationship was found over the entire concentration range.
To check the accuracy of the calibration a sample containing 0.27% w/v was
included; 0.26% w/v was found.

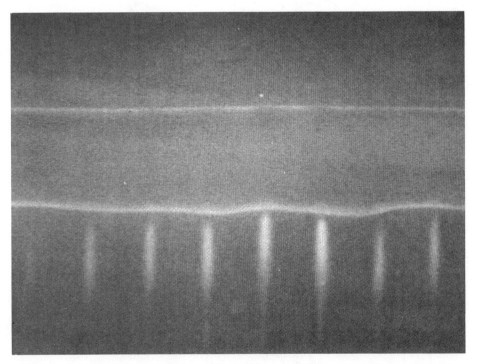

Fig. 1. Unprocessed image of aryl sulphonate separated from base oil.

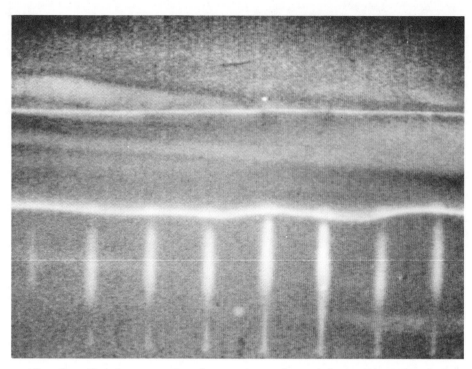

Fig. 2. Signal averaged and contrast enhanced image from Figure 1.

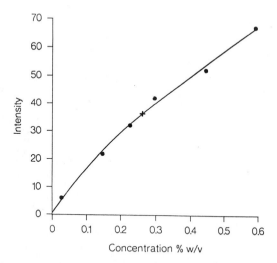

Fig. 3. Calibration obtained from spot intensities in Figure 2. The line
is a polynomial fit (of order 3). The point marked + is the 0.27%
w/v test sample.

To test the effectiveness of the technique with 'real industrial
samples' a separation of a number of detergents in lubricating oil was
carried out. The normal video image obtained is shown in Figure 4. The
fluorescing spots due to the sulphonates are barely discernible. The image
acquired using the integration procedure is shown in Figure 5.

The bright spots corresponding to the sulphonates can be clearly seen. Additionally, a number of dark spots become apparent. These are due to phenates and cationic surfactants, also present in the sample, which quench the background fluorescence of the F254 plates.

In Figure 6 a sequence of images obtained from the same plate at 5, 10, 15 and 25 minutes after dipping in pinacryptol yellow solution is shown. This clearly shows the fluorescence intensity increasing to a maximum after approximately 10 minutes, after which it rapidly decays. The reason for this is believed to be due to the degradation of the pinacryptol yellow ion-pair by the active silica substrate. Attempts to regenerate the fluorescence, by redipping the plate in pinacryptol yellow, resulted in even further deterioration of the image.

CONCLUSIONS

We have shown that by using an image integration technique high quality images can be obtained from weakly fluorescing compounds separated on HPTLC plates.

Phenates and other surfactants which cause quenching of the background fluorescence can also be detected at very low concentrations. Quantitative analysis can then be carried out by a variety of image processing techniques. The limits of detection are well below that required for the analysis of aryl sulphonate detergents in many industrial oils.

The image processing system allows images of the entire plate to be acquired very rapidly. Thus to acquire and average 800 images from a fluorescent plate took only 33 seconds. This not only provides faster 'sample throughput' but more importantly, quantitative analysis of unstable

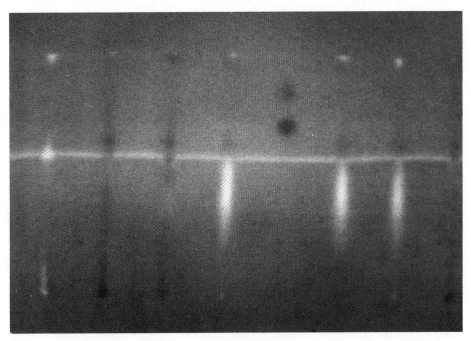

Fig. 4. Unprocessed image of detergent package separated from lubricating oil.

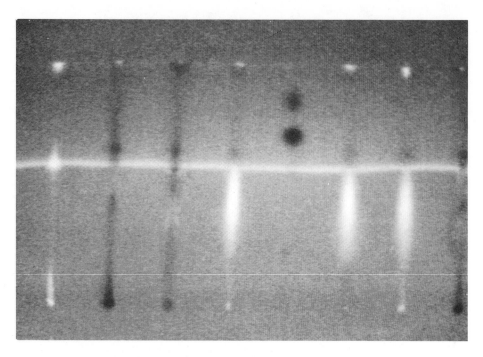

Fig. 5. Processed image from Figure 4.

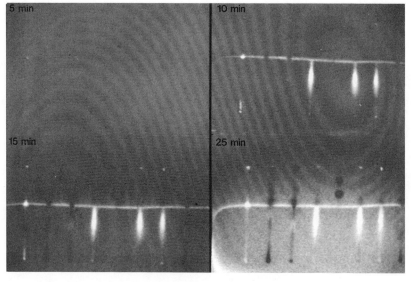

Fig. 6. Successive processed images captured during the development –
         decay cycle of the detergent package.

compounds can be achieved. Speed was shown to be of critical importance in
the analysis of sulphonate/pinacryptol yellow adducts, where within ten
minutes the fluorescent intensity had dramatically changed. To obtain the
same level of quantitative information with a densitometer, using the
zig-zag scanning mode, would take in the order of 30 minutes.

ACKNOWLEDGEMENT

The Authors wish to thank the Management of the British Petroleum Company plc for permission to publish this paper.

REFERENCES

1. R. M. Belchamber, H. Read, and J. D. M. Roberts, Planar Chromat.-ography, Vol. 1, R. E. Kaiser, ed., Heuthig Publishing Company, Heidelberg, p. 207, (1986).

2. R. M. Belchamber, H. Read, and J. D. M. Roberts, J.Chromatogr., 395:47 (1987).

3. T. Devenyi, Acta.Biochim.Biophys.Hungh.Acad., 11:1 (1976).

4. J. Kramer, N. B. Gusev, and P. Friedrich, Anal.Biochem., 108:295 (1980).

5. B. F. Aycock, D. E. Weil, D. V. Sinicropi, and D. L. McIlwain, Comput.Biomed.Res., 14:314 (1981).

6. S. Pongor, J.Liquid Chromatogr., 5:1583 (1982).

7. P. A. Jansson, L. B. Grim, J. G. Elias, E. A. Bagley, and K. K. Lonberg-Holm, Electrophoresis, 4:82 (1983).

8. S. P. Spragg, M. I. Jones, and B. J. Hill, Anal.Biochem., 129:255 (1983).

9. T. Manabe and T. Okuyama, J.Chromatogr., 264:435 (1983).

10. R. P. Tracey, and D. S. Young, Clin.Chem., 30:462 (1984).

11. W. Woiwode, GIT Fachz Lab., 114:498 (1984).

12. M. Prosek, A. Medja, M. Katic, Instrumental HPTLC., Published by Inst. for Chromatography, Bad Durkheim (1985).

13. T. S. Ford-Holevinski and N. S. Radin, Anal.Biochem., 150:359 (1985).

14. D. D. Rees, K. E. Fogarty, L. K. Levy, F. S. Fay, Anal.Biochem., 144:461 (1985).

15. S. Bardocz, T. Karsai, and P. Elodi, Chromatographia, 20:23 (1985).

16. M. L. Gianelli, J. B. Callis, N. H. Andersen, and G. D. Christian, Anal.Chem., 53:1357 (1981).

17. M. Prosek, M. Medja, J. Korsic, M. Pristav, and R. E. Kaiser, Planar Chromatography, Vol. 1, R. E. Kaiser, ed., Heuthig Publishing Company, Heidelberg, p. 221 (1986).

18. M. L. Gianelli, D. H. Burns, J. B. Callis, G. D. Christian, and N. H. Andersen, Anal.Chem., 55:1858 (1983).

19. D. H. Burns, J. B. Callis, and G. D. Christian, Trends in Anal Chem., 5:50 (1986).

ANALYTICAL ROTATION PLANAR CHROMATOGRAPHY

Sz. Nyiredy,* K. Dallenbach-Toelke and O. Sticher

Pharmazeutisches Institut
Eidgenössische Technische Hochschule Zürich (ETH)
CH-8092 Zurich, Switzerland

SUMMARY

A new analytical rotation planar chromatographic method, micro chamber rotation planar chromatography (M-RPC), is described in detail and compared with ultra-micro chamber rotation planar chromatography (U-RPC). The principle and possibilities of these forced-flow methods are discussed with respect to the chamber types, applicable stationary and mobile phases, development modes and operating parameters.

In the micro chamber the vapor space is variable whilst in the ultra-micro chamber it is practically eliminated; therefore, M-RPC resembles a saturated system while U-RPC is more akin to an unsaturated system. The mobile phase has to be optimized accordingly and can then be transferred from thin-layer chromatography (TLC) preassays to M-RPC or U-RPC without modification. All commercially available stationary phases can be used for the separations using either TLC or high-performance (HP) TLC quality. Circular, anticircular, and linear development modes and combinations thereof are possible using both methods.

The advantages and disadvantages of both M-RPC and U-RPC are discussed and compared with other planar chromatographic methods.

INTRODUCTION

Since the introduction of the term "Thin-Layer Chromatography" by Stahl in 1956[1] the use of the technique has expanded dynamically[2,3]. For a long time thin-layer chromatographic separations were achieved only by capillary action. More recently forced-flow methods have been introduced.

The first forced-flow planar chromatographic technique was achieved using centrifugal force[4]. From centrifugally-accelerated paper chromatography centrifugal thin-layer chromatography was developed[5]. Centrifugal layer chromatography (CLC)[6,7] as a circular on-line preparative

---

* Visiting scientist on leave from Semmelweis Medical University, Institute of Pharmacognosy, H-1085 Budapest, Hungary.

method has gained importance in the separation and isolation of naturally
occurring compounds. In CLC the layer rotates in a stationary chamber
which results in evaporation of large amounts of the mobile phase during
the chromatographic process. This has a number of adverse effects, including the "surface" effect, the "standing front" effect, and a change in the
mobile phase composition[8,9]. These adverse effects have, until now, made
the application of centrifugal force for analytical separations practically
impossible.

In 1978 Tyihák et al.,[10] introduced the first modern analytical
forced-flow planar chromatographic method using a pressurized chamber.
From this concept overpressure layer chromatography (OPLC)[11-13] was
developed. OPLC makes it possible to use HPTLC plates over a longer separation distance than 5 cm without a loss in resolution. In OPLC the linear
and continuous development modes are generally used, but circular development is also possible. At present two OPLC chamber types (Chrompres-10 and
25) exist where 10 or 25 bar pressure is applied.

Recently, high pressure planar liquid chromatography (HPPLC) has been
reported by Kaiser[14] as a new analytical technique. In HPPLC a pressure
of 80 bar or more may be applied for rapid circular development. More
recently the term rotation planar chromatography (RPC) has been introduced,
because, in general usage, CLC stands for column liquid chromatography
rather than for centrifugal layer chromatography.

Depending on the chamber types and techniques used in RPC, five
different methods may be applied: normal chamber RPC (N-RPC), micro chamber
RPC (M-RPC), ultra-micro chamber RPC (U-RPC)[15], as well as sequential RPC
(S-RPC)[16] (until now named as sequential centrifugal layer chromatography, SCLC), and column RPC (C-RPC)[17] (until now named as centrifugal
planar-column chromatography, CPCC).

We will now present the two new analytical RPC methods (M-RPC and
U-RPC) and compare these methods with other planar chromatographic
techniques.

EXPERIMENTAL

Description of M-RPC

M-RPC is a centrifugally-accelerated planar chromatographic technique
in a special chamber where the vapor space is reduced and can be varied;
therefore, M-RPC resembles a saturated system. The co-rotating annular
chromatographic chamber (Figure 2) is, in effect, closed. The quartz cover
plate (1 in Figure 2) of the chamber is fixed in a ring in the upper part
of the chamber. The distance between the chromatographic layer (4 in
Figure 2) and the glass may be varied by a supporting ring (5 in Figure 2).

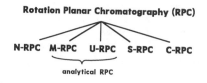

Fig. 1. Rotation planar chromatographic methods.

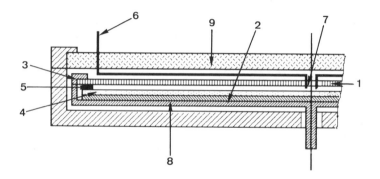

Fig. 2. Cross sectional view of M-RPC. (See text for detailed description).

For solvent delivery, a hole (6 in Figure 2) is located in the center of
the cover plate. Due to the centrifugal force and the capillary action,
the eluent migrates through the stationary phase.

After the prepared plate is fitted into the lower part of the chamber
(8 in Figure 2), the latter is closed by a ring (3 in Figure 2) that is
fixed on the quartz glass with a sealing ring and attached by screws. The
outer lid (9 in Figure 2) of the instrument is then shut, one of the
horizontally and vertically variable solvent delivery systems is placed
through the hole of the quartz glass, and on the rotating layer the
separation may then be started with an adequate mobile phase.

Description of U-RPC

The construction of the co-rotating chamber in U-RPC is similar to
M-RPC with the difference that the space between the quartz glass cover
plate and the layer is eliminated by a suitable silicon plate that is
placed under the layer. So in U-RPC, the vapor space is practically
eliminated; therefore, U-RPC is similar to an unsaturated system[15].

Choice of Operating Conditions

In addition to the stationary and mobile phases used, the rotation
speed and the development mode are the most important parameters in analytical RPC.

For M-RPC and U-RPC, all commercially available precoated plates (20 x
20cm, 10 x 20cm, 10 x 10cm) of TLC and HPTLC quality may be used. In both
methods, the mobile phase velocity may be varied with the rotation speed,
which is continuously regulated between 100 and 1500 rpm. The more the
rotation speed is increased, the faster is the migration of the mobile
phase, as shown in Figure 3.

The optimal rotary velocity depends on the separation problem. The
flow rate is limited by the amount of solvent that may be kept in the layer
without it floating over the surface[8]. The greater the amount of applied
solvent, the higher the rotation speed has to be in order to keep the
mobile phase within the layer. The amount of migrating solvent may also be
increased by scratching a round hole in the center of the layer, whose
perimeter may be varied according to the optimal mobile phase velocity[15].

The velocity of the mobile phase in the sorbent may also be varied
locally by scraping pathways of various forms in the layer. With these
special preparations of the plate, the linear and anticircular development

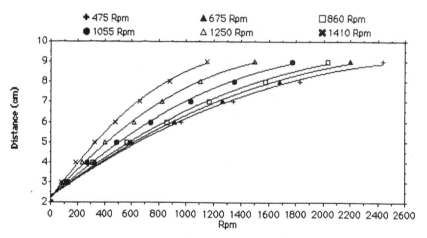

Fig. 3. Mobile phase velocity and its dependence of the rotation speed.

modes are made possible[15]. All development modes may be combined, depending on the separation problem. Some of the possible combinations are
depicted in Figure 4. Combinations of circular and anticircular development are shown in Figure 4 a and 4b. These are used to improve resolution,
reduce band broadening, and simplify quantitative determinations. In
Figure 4c a combination of circular, linear, and circular modes is shown.
shown.

     It must be remembered that in the anticircular mode and its combi-
nations, the pathway gets smaller and quantitative determination may become
increasingly difficult near the outside of the plate. If no satisfactory
separation is achieved in the middle and/or lower Rf ranges with the mobile
phase used, a certain type of sequential technique[15], can be employed in
M-RPC and U-RPC. After the chromatographic run, these substances are
pushed back to the start with a strong solvent at a low rotation speed.
This is done with the vertically and horizontally variable solvent delivery
system while the micro or ultra-micro chamber is opened. After drying the
plate with inert gas, the separation of these substances can be started
again with another suitable mobile phase. The separation distance and
number of samples depend on the development mode. In circular development,
up to 30 samples may be applied on a 20cm diameter plate with an 8cm
development. Because of the relation $Rf_{circ} = Rf_{lin}^2$[18], in a stationary
chamber the sample would be applied in the center of the plate. The Δ Rf
values of the separated compounds would, therefore, be greater in the lower
Rf range and smaller in the higher Rf range. If the samples were to be
applied on an r-cm diameter circle for analytical separation, the relation

$$Rf_{circ} = \sqrt{Rf_{lin}(1 + 2r) + r^2} - r$$

is valid. The longer the distance r (r>2cm) is, consequently the circular
Rf values of the separated compounds are more similar to the linear Rf
values. In analytical RPC improved resolution can be achieved because the
mobile phase velocity can be increased by centrifugal force (see Figure 3)
and varied locally, which is the result of the differing types of
separation pathways (see Figure 4). The number of samples that can be
applied is reduced (between 4 to 12) in anticircular and linear development
modes and their combinations. In the linear development mode samples may
be applied either as spots or bands. For both M-RPC and U-RPC all mobile
phases previously optimized on TLC plates can be transferred directly
without further modification as follows.

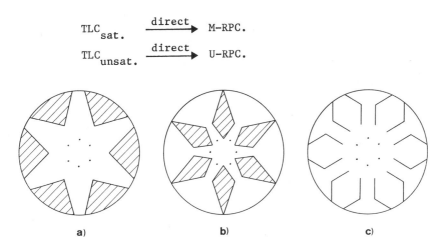

$$TLC_{sat.} \xrightarrow{\text{direct}} M\text{-}RPC.$$

$$TLC_{unsat.} \xrightarrow{\text{direct}} U\text{-}RPC.$$

a)   b)   c)

Fig. 4. Preparation of TLC plates for various development modes in M-RPC.
(a) Combination of the circular and anticircular modes.
(b) Combination of the anticircular and circular modes.
(c) Combination of circular, linear, and circular modes.

In the case where the mobile phase for the separation of apolar compounds
was optimized in an unsaturated chamber and the M-RPC technique is used
then the solvent strength has to be reduced. The separation of polar
compounds obtained with an unsaturated TLC system may only be transferred
to M-RPC following modification of the solvent composition, since the
composition of the multi-component mobile phase is changed due to the
effects of evaporation[20]. Mobile phase optimization may be achieved
systematically with the "PRISMA" model[21,22], which combines the solvent
strength and selectivity in a three dimensional design. The separation of
colored compounds may be observed during the chromatographic process
through the instrument. UV active compounds may be seen with a built-in UV
lamp through the quartz cover plate of the chambers at 254 nm or 366 nm.
This allows the in-process control of the separation and is one of the
basic requirements for the sequential technique. Temperature may also be
held constant during the separation.

Materials and Methods

Opium alkaloids were obtained from Roth (Karlsruhe, FRG.). The
furocoumarins and ginsenosides were isolated and identified at the Institute of Pharmacy, ETH Zurich. Samples were applied with a Linomat III TLC
spotter with a 1mm band width or with a modified Nanomat spotter, both from
Camag (Muttenz, Switzerland). All solvents were analytical grade.

The TLC preassays, for mobile phase optimization, were carried out on
silica 60 F_{254} TLC alufoils (Merck, Darmstadt, FRG.) in unsaturated
chambers for U-RPC separations[23] and in saturated chambers for M-RPC
separations. Both types of RPC separations were carried out on silica 60
F_{254} HPTLC alufoils (Merck, Darmstadt).

For the separations, the ROTACHROM rotation planar chromatograph
(Petazon AG, Zug, Switzerland) was employed. The corners of the plates
were cut off[15]. The separation distance was 8cm, and samples were applied in the form of spots on a 4cm diameter circle around the center of
the plate.

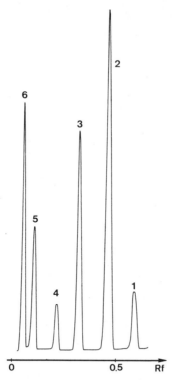

Fig. 5. M-RPC separation of opium alkaloids. 1 - noscapine, 2 -
papaverine, 3 - thebaine, 4 - morphine, 5 - codeine, 6 - narceine
(conditions see text).

For visual detection of the ginsenosides, 1% vanillin sulfuric acid
was used. Densitograms were taken at 254 nm for the opium alkaloids, at
295 nm for the furocoumarins and at 540 nm for the ginsenosides with a
Shimadzu 920 scanner (Shimadzu, Kyoto, Japan) or with a TLC scanner 11 from
Camag (Muttenz, Switzerland).

RESULTS

M-RPC-Separation of Opium Alkaloids

The six main alkaloids of Papaver somniferum were separated on HPTLC
plates in a saturated chamber with a mobile phase of tetrahydrofuran,
hexane 3:1 with 3% diethylamine as modifier (mobile phase 1) with good
resolution. However, narceine stayed at the spot origin. When ethanol was
used with 3% diethylamine (mobile phase 2), narceine had an Rf value of
0.45, but the separation of the other compounds in the mixture was not
satisfactory; therefore, the M-RPC separation was carried out with solvent
delivery system 1 and mobile phase 1 for a distance of 6.5cm, then mobile
phase 2 was applied continously with solvent delivery system 11. The
separation was continously observed at 254 nm. The resulting separation is
shown in Figure 5 with all six alkaloids baseline resolved.

U-RPC - Separation of Furocoumarin Isomers

The five main furocoumarin isomers from Heracleum sphondylium were
separated on a HPTLC plate with a 5cm separation distance in an unsaturated

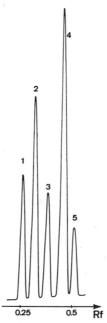

Fig. 6. U-RPC separation of furocoumarin isomers. 1 - sphondin, 2 -
iso-pimpinellin, 3 - bergapten, 4 - pimpinellin, 5 - iso-bergapten
(conditions see text).

chamber. The mobile phase was optimized with the "PRISMA" model and
transferred to U-RPC without modification. The densitogram of the U-RPC
separation at 8cm separation distance is given in Figure 6. All five
furocoumarin isomers were separated with an excellent resolution.

M-RPC and U-RPC Separation of Ginsenosides

The TLC separations were carried out in saturated and unsaturated
chambers. The best separation was obtained with a mobile phase composition
of methyl ethyl ketone-methanol-water-hexane. In the saturated chamber the
ratio was 80:10:10:15 v/v (mobile phase 1) and in the unsaturated chamber
70:22:8:30 v/v (mobile phase 2).

The M-RPC-separation (Figure 7a) was obtained with mobile phase 1, and
the U-RPC-separation (Figure 7b) with mobile phase 2. The U-RPC separation
was better in the higher Rf range, therefore, no baseline separation could
be achieved between Rb1 and Rb2. With M-RPC all substances were baseline
separated.

DISCUSSION

Characterization and Comparison of the Methods

The most important parameter used to compare different planar chromatographic methods is the forced flow, which influences the separation. A
comparison of the migration of the mobile phase front as function of time
for a distance between 3 and 10cm is shown in Figure 8.

Comparing the functions of both completely closed systems, the function is almost linear for OPLC in linear development mode, for circular

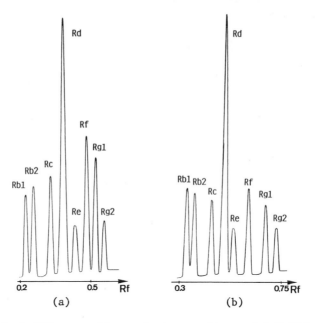

Fig. 7. Analytical RPC separations of ginsenosides. (a) M-RPC separation (conditions see text). (b) U-RPC separation (conditions see text).

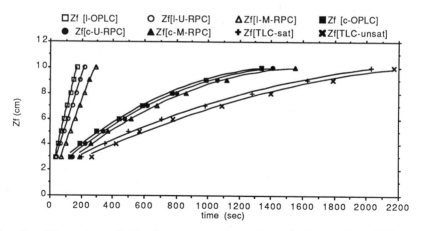

Fig. 8. Migration of the front as a function of time using different planar chromatographic methods.

OPLC it is a curved function, because the volume of the stationary phase increases along the radius. For linear U-RPC the function is slightly flatter than for linear OPLC, for linear M-RPC as a saturated system, the migration of the front is even slower. For circular development the relation between these three techniques is similar. In linear development the flow is faster on TLC plates in saturated systems than in unsaturated chambers. However, in both cases the migration is slower than with circular forced-flow techniques. To the best of our knowledge, no chamber for circular or anticircular analytical TLC exists with a migration distance longer than 5cm, so these methods were not considered in the comparison. Both types of forced-flow planar chromatographic techniques (OPLC and RPC) have certain limitations. In OPLC that limitation depends on the applied pressure, which confines the applied mobile phase velocity, in RPC it depends on the amount of solvent the layer may take at the rotation speed applied. In both cases, the limitation also depends on the viscosity of the mobile phase.

Comparing analytical OPLC with RPC, RPC has advantage that separations may be carried out with or without the influence of solvent vapor which may be important in certain cases (e.g., for the separation of alkaloids). The major problem in OPLC, the disturbing zone[24], which distorts the separation and makes evaluation impossible, does not exist for M-RPC and U-RPC because they are not completely closed chromatographic systems.

In both new methods quantitative determination is easier because, unlike OPLC, the multi-front effect[25] generally does not appear. If the separations are carried out with multi-component mobile phases, the fronts of the different solvents may be observed in OPLC as small lines shown in Figure 9, on the plate and in the diagram. Although the properties of U-RPC are similar to OPLC, since U-RPC is not a completely closed system, the front effect is rarely observed, therefore, the corners of the characteristic are slightly rounded. The more saturated a system is the smaller is this effect (Figure 9) and, therefore, the influence on the quantitative determination is less.

Advantages and Disadvantages of Analytical RPC

Both types of RPC have many advantages: first, they are forced-flow techniques and, therefore, fine particle size plates with all kinds of materials can be used without loss of resolution in a separation distance between 8 and 11cm. All mobile phases, from saturated or unsaturated TLC systems, may be applied for M-RPC or U-RPC, respectively. Because neither are completely closed systems, the disturbing zone and the multi-front effect do not distort either the separation or determinations.

Another benefit is that the mobile phase velocity can be varied with the rotation speed, as well as the perimeter of the solvent application in the center of the plate. The circular, anticircular, and linear development modes and their combinations can be used and, consequently, the mobile phase velocity can be varied locally.

During the chromatography the separation may be observed at 254 and 366 nm, so a gradient may be carried out with the solvent delivery system

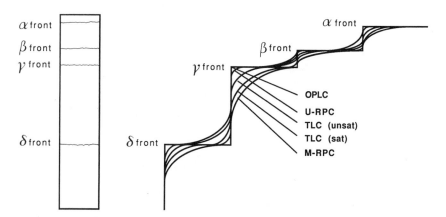

Fig. 9.   Characteristics of the multi-front effect using different planar chromatographic methods.

without stopping the run. This also enables a type of sequential technique to be used.

The analytical M-RPC and U-RPC separations may be scaled up to preparative purposes, which is of importance as an isolation technique.

The main disadvantage of these methods is that the applied parameters of the system (rotation speed, perimeter of the solvent application, development mode) have to be considered for the rate at which solvent is delivered otherwise the mobile phase flows on top of the applied sample and the layer, or the effect of the standing front may occur[8]. In the circular and anticircular development modes and their combinations quantitative determination may sometimes be difficult with the densitometers currently available.

The new analytical forced-flow planar chromatographic methods M-RPC and U-RPC offer many options (e.g., choice of vapor volume size, stationary phase, mobile phase, isocratic or gradient elution, development technique). They have been shown to be very versatile in the instrumental high performance separation of various naturally occurring compounds and synthetic products.

ACKNOWLEDGEMENT

A research grant from the Swiss National Science Foundation is gratefully acknowledged.

REFERENCES

1. E. Stahl, Pharmazie, 11:633 (1956).
2. A. Zlatkis and R. E. Kaiser, eds., in: "HPTLC - High Performance Thin-Layer Chromatography," Elsevier, Amsterdam, New York, (1977).
3. W. Bertsch, S. Hara, R. E. Kaiser and A. Zlatkis, eds., Instrumental HPTLC, Huethig, Heidelberg, (1980).
4. Z. Deyl, J. Rosmus and M. Pavlicek, Chromatogr.Rev. 6:19 (1964).
5. G. Caronna, Chim.Ind.(Milan) 37:113 (1955),
6. E. Heftmann, J. M. Krochta, D. F. Farkas and S. Schwimmer, J.Chromatogr., 66:365 (1972).
7. K. Hostettmann, M. Hostettmann-Kaldas and O. Sticher, J.Chromatogr., 202:154 (1980).
8. Sz. Nyiredy, S. Y. Mészáros, K. Nyiredy-Mikita, K. Dallenbach-Tölke and O. Sticher, GIT Suppl.Chromatogr., No. 3:51 (1986).
9. Sz. Nyiredy, K. Nyiredy-Mikita, S. Y. Mészáros, K. Dallenbach-Tölke and O. Sticher, Planta Med., 425 (1986).
10. E. Tyihák, H. Kalász, E. Mincsovics and J. Nagy, Proc.17th Hung.Ann. Meet.Biochem., Kecskemét, Abstr.pp. 49-50 (1977); C. A. 88 15386 u (1978).
11. E. Tyihák, E. Mincsovics and H. Kalász, J.Chromatogr., 174:75 (1979).
12. E. Mincsovics, E. Tyihák and H. Kalász, J.Chromatogr., 191:293 (1980).
13. E. Tyihák, E. Mincsovics, H. Kalász and J. Nagy, J.Chromatogr., 211:45 (1981).
14. R. E. Kaiser "HPPLC" (Planar Chromatography Volume II) Huethig, Heidelberg, (1987).
15. Sz. Nyiredy, S.Y. Mészáros, K. Dallenbach-Toelke, K. Nyiredy-Mikita and O. Sticher, J.Planar Chromatogr., submitted for publication.
16. Sz. Nyiredy, C. A. J. Erdelmeier and O. Sticher, in: "Planar Chromatography," Vol. 1, R. E. Kaiser, ed., Huethig, Heidelberg, pp. 119-164, (1986).

17. Sz. Nyiredy, S. Y. Mészáros, K. Nyiredy-Mikita, K. Dallenbach-Toelke and O. Sticher, J.High Resolut.Chromatogr., Chromatogr.Commun., 9:605 (1986).
18. R. E. Kaiser, J.High Resolut.Chromatogr.,Chromatogr.Commun., 1:164 (1978).
19. G. Geiss, in: "Die Parameter der Dünnschicht-Chromatographie," Friedrich Vieweg & Sohn, Braunschweig, pp. 45-46 (1972).
20. Sz. Nyiredy, C. A. J. Erdelmeier, B. Meier and O. Sticher, GIT Suppl. Chromatogr., No. 4:24 (1985).
21. Sz. Nyiredy, C. A. J. Erdelmeier, B. Meier and O. Sticher, Planta Medica, 241 (1985).
22. K. Dallenbach-Toelke, Sz. Nyiredy, B. Meier and O. Sticher, J.Chromatogr., 365:63 (1986).
23. K. Dallenbach-Tölke, Ph.D. thesis No. 8178, ETH Zurich, (1986).
24. Sz. Nyiredy, S. Y. Mészáros, K. Dallenbach-Toelke, K. Nyiredy-Mikita and O. Sticher, J.High Resolut.Chromatogr.Chromatogr.Commun., 10:352 (1987).
25. Sz. Nyiredy, C. A. J. Erdelmeier and O. Sticher, in: "Proceedings on TLC With Special Emphasis on Overpressured Layer Chromatography (OPLC)," E. Tyihák, ed., Labor MIM, Budapest, pp. 222-231 (1986).

ANALYTICAL AND PREPARATIVE OVERPRESSURED

LAYER CHROMATOGRAPHY (OPLC)

Emil Mincsovics* and E. Tyihák**

*Labor MIM, H-1445, Budapest, P O Box 280, Hungary
**Plant. Prot. Inst., Hungarian Academy of Sciences
H-1525, Budapest, P O Box 102, Hungary

SUMMARY

Aspects of the use of overpressured layer chromatography (OPLC) as an instrumentalised version of planar liquid chromatography, suitable for both analytical and preparative off-line and on-line separations, are described.

For example the eluent strength and solvent composition considerably influence the applicability of off-line OPLC owing to the demixing of the solvent during chromatography. The disturbing effect due to this demixing phenomenon can be reduced or eliminated if the differences in solvent strength between the eluent constitutents are kept to a minimum.

There is a strong correlation between dry and wet OPLC separations regarding retention characteristics, which offers a new prospect for the modelling of high performance liquid chromatography.

In the case of preparative on-line separation and detection prewetting the stationary phase from outlet side can eliminate disturbances which otherwise adversely affect detection.

INTRODUCTION

Overpressured layer chromatography (OPLC) is a collective term for techniques using a pressurized ultramicro chamber, a pump system for the delivery of the eluent into a chamber containing modified analytical and preparative chromatoplates under pressure. The basic ancestor of this technique is the ultramicro (UM) chamber[1] from which we developed the experimental pressurized UM chamber where an external pressure was applied to the sorbent layer surface by means of a cushion system. In this way it was possible to apply an overpressure to the eluent to force it through the sorbent bed[2,3,4]. Based on experiences with the experimental pressurized UM chambers, the Labor Instrumental Works (Budapest-Esztergom, Hungary) developed the CHROMPRES 10 and CHROMPRES 25, which became the first commercially available OPLC instruments. As in traditional thin-layer and high performance thin-layer chromatography (TLC/HPTLC), every kind of development can be performed in OPLC including circular, anticircular, triangular, one and two directional linear and two dimensional[2-6]. In addition it is also possible to develop more than one layer simultaneously in over-pressured multi-layer chromatography (OPMLC), and thus multiply the sample throughput of the OPLC system[7].

To increase the resolution in the case of a selective solvent system and compounds running with low Rf values it is possible to run using longer or continuous development techniques[3,6,8,9]. Multiple development has also been combined with continuous development[10].

In off-line OPLC all the principal steps in the chromatographic process, such as sample application, separation, quantitative evaluation and/or isolation are performed as separate operations. In the on-line mode it is possible to measure the solutes in the eluting solvent by connecting the flow-cell of a detector to the solvent outlet. The entire chromatographic process can be performed on-line by connecting a loop injector to the solvent inlet and UV detector to the solvent outlet, in much the same way as in HPLC[11]. In this system different combinations of on-line and off-line steps can also be employed.

Here we present some new aspects of our work in the field of analytical and preparative off-line and on-line OPLC.

EXPERIMENTAL

Apparatus

OPLC instruments (CHROMPRES 10 and CHROMPRES 25) were fitted with two eluent connections and were obtained from Labor MIM (Budapest, Hungary). One of the eluent connections was used as an inlet and the other was used for an outlet. The inlet was connected with a loop injector and the outlet was coupled to a Liqudet 308 UV detector (Labor MIM) having 8µl cell volume.

The distance between the inlet and outlet was 180mm, i.e. the distance between eluent directing troughs on the teflon insert sheet. The width of these eluent directing troughs was 0.8mm and these were selected according to the width of the plate used.

The inner diameter of the original inlet and outlet was reduced by inserting 0.25mm I.D. tubes into them. Sample application was carried out in the off-line mode directly onto the dry layer using either Hamilton microsyringes or a Linomat III (Camag, Muttenz, Switzerland). In the on-line mode samples were applied to dry or wet plates, by a loop injector. Quantitative evaluation was accomplished by a SHIMADZU CS 920 scanning densitometer (Shimadzu, Kyoto, Japan).

Chemicals

The sorbent layers used were TLC (5554), HPTLC (5548) and preparative TLC (13794), the last with a concentrating zone, silica gel chromatoplates obtained from E. Merck & Co. (Darmstadt, F.R.G.). These were pretreated by sealing on all four sides by means of an impregnation process which was performed using the IMPRES UP polymer suspension (Labor MIM).

Solvents used were LiChrosolv (Merck) and reagent-grade. Xanthines were purchased from Merck Co. and poppy alkaloids were supplied by the Alkaloida Chemical Works (Tiszavasvári, Hungary). The dyes used were test dye mixture I and II (Camag) and Fat red. Samples were dissolved in the solvent used for chromatography.

RESULTS AND DISCUSSION

Classical OPLC is an off-line system because sample application, chromatographic development, quantitative evaluation and/or preparative isolation are carried out independently of one another. It is obvious that there are some advantages of the off-line system in planar liquid chromatography as, in general, several samples can be processed in parallel and only the spots of analytical interest need be assessed. In addition quantitative evaluation can be repeated with different detection parameters and there is also the possibility of the visual evaluation of spots or bands obtained. We believe that these advantages, when combined with the special merits of OPLC, result in a similar advance in the field of planar liquid chromatography as was seen earlier with the introduction of the development of HPLC in the field of column chromatography.

In the case of CHROMPRES 25 it is possible to continually remove the eluent allowing the technique to perform continuous development thereby increasing the resolution on the layer. Providing that none of the components of interest are lost in the drained eluent the components of interest can either be detected <u>in-situ</u> by densitometry or can be isolated from the layer using classical methods. By connecting a flow-cell detector to the outlet is is possible to measure solutes eluting in the eluent. Sample application can be carried out either off-line or on-line by connecting a suitable injector to the inlet. Thus, this system has high

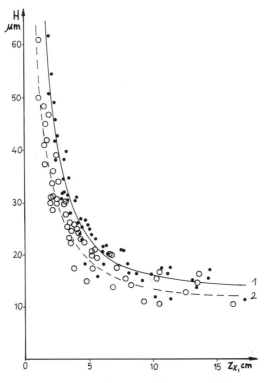

Fig. 1. Effect of the migration distance on HETP values using full off-line and on-line injection methods. External pressure on membrane, 2.5 MPa; eluent, toluene; temperature 27°C; eluent front velocity, 1.67 cm/min; layer, HPTLC silica gel 60; samples, dye mixture ($0.8 < R_f < 0.1$). 1, on-line injection-separation system ——— ; 2, full off-line system --- .

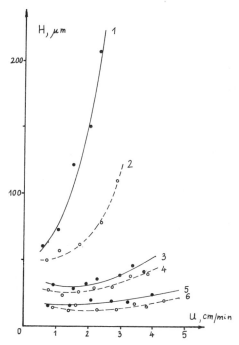

Fig. 2. Effect of the solvent front velocity on HETP values using full
off-line and full on-line OPLC. Eternal pressure on membrane, 2.5
MPa; eluent, 150-octane-THF 93:7, v/v; temperature 28°C; migration
distances in full off-line system, 174-177 mm; bed length in full
on-line system, 180 mm; sample, Fat red. 1-2, PLC; 3-4, TLC; 5-6,
HPTLC layers; dotted line, full off-line system.

flexibility and different combinations of the various on-line and off-line
procedures can also be used covering the region between full off-line and
full on-line OPLC.

As was found in the field of HPLC, and also our first results with
on-line OPLC, the extra-column band broadening depended on the volume, size
and form of the connections. In the case of the on-line CHROMPRES system
band broadening can be reduced by using narrower directing troughs and
connection tubes of reduced diameter fitting into the inlet and outlet
tubes.

It was found in full off-line OPLC that the HETP values are not
independent of the migration distance of different components[11] and
decrease considerably with migration distances. As in HPLC the number of
theoretical plates increases linearly with column length ($N=L/H$)[12,13] and
the plate number is additive using connected columns[14]. These assume
constant HETP values. The results shown in Figure 1 demonstrate the effect
of the migration distance on HETP values using full off-line OPLC and the
on-line injection-separation system in which the injection occurs onto a
completely wetted layer. In both cases the band width was determined using
a densitometer. It can be seen that curves are very similar, but the
on-line injected system gives higher HETP values. The source of this
difference between the two systems lies in the extra-column band broadening, which does not occur in the off-line system. These curves show that,
over a limited bed length and migration distance, the HETP values become
practically constant as was found in HPLC[12-14].

60

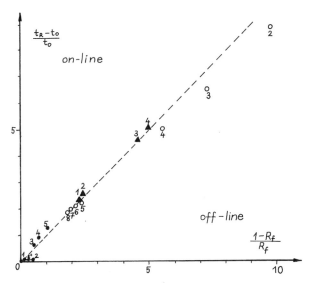

Fig. 3. Relationship between off-line and on-line OPLC retentions on
silica. ▲ eluent, n-heptane; samples 1, phenanthrene; 2, pyrene;
3, chrysene; 4, perylene. ● eluent CH_2Cl_2-CH_3CH_2OH, 100:10 v/v,
samples 1, Fat red; 2, butter yellow; 3, caffeine; 4,
theophylline; 5, theobromine. ○ eluent $CHCl_3$-CH_3CN-CH_3CH_2COOH-
H_2O, 52:5:20:25:2.5 v/v, samples 2, normorphine; 3, narceine; 4,
codeine; 5, narcotoline; 6, thebaine; 7, papaverine; 8, narcotine.

This extra-column band broadening also occurs at the outlet side when
full on-line OPLC is used. The effect of linear front velocity on HETP
values can be seen in Figure 2 using different chromatoplates for full
off-line and full on-line OPLC separations.

In order to allow a direct comparison between the off and on line
systems the migration distance of the spot in the off-line system, and the
bed length of the on-line system were the same. In addition the original
band size and directing trough width were identical for both methods. The
difference between these two systems is therefore due to the extra-column
band broadening which is very difficult to reduce below a reasonable
limit[13].

In the case of OPLC separations using dry sorbent layers we have to
take into account the following main phenomena: the wetness of the sorbent
layer, the phenomenon of chromatographic solvent demixing and the balance
between the mobile and stationary phases.

The first part of the development is the pre-wetting period which
lasts until the eluent front (F) reaches the outlet (this corresponds to
conventional OPLC). On the layer partially and perfectly wetted zones can
be observed. This phenomenon occurs whether single or multi-component
eluents are used. Another problem which arises with adsorption, as well as
reversed-phase developments occurs when the eluent system has solvents of
different strength. These are sorbed differently by the sorbent sites and
this results in the formation of secondary solvent fronts[15]. These
fronts divide the sorbent layer into zones of different eluting strength,
within which the solvent polarity is practically the same, whilst at the
fronts themselves there is a sudden increasing in solvent polarity giving
rise to "polarity steps".

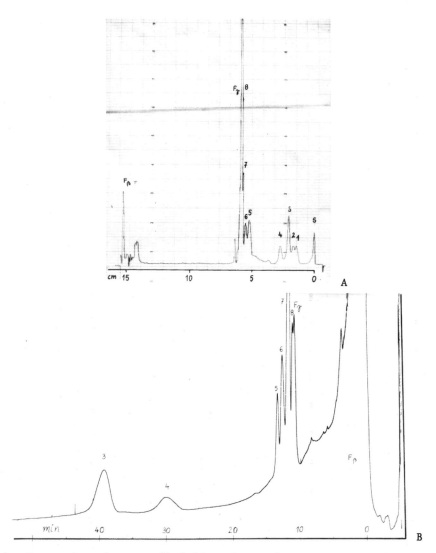

Fig. 4.   Separation of poppy alkaloids. External pressure on membrane, 2.5
MPa, eluent, chloroform–acetonitrile–propionic acid–water,
52.5:20:25:2.5 v/v, front velocity 2.61 cm/min, temperature 20°C,
detection at 254 nm. Samples, 1, morphine; 2, normorphine; 3,
narceine; 4, codeine; 5, narcotoline; 6, thebaine; 7, papaverine;
8, narcotine. A – full off-line process; B – off-line sample
application and on-line separation–detection.

        Having left the layer the eluent appears in the detector where it may
contain bubbles which can cause detection problems. This can be solved in
practice by prewetting from the outlet direction until the eluent front
reaches the point of sample application, followed by conventional development using the eluent inlet. Using this mode of separation the bulk of the
air is removed from the layer prior to development. The residual air
remaining in the sorbent bed will be partially dissolved in the eluent and
will not cause further difficulties. Using this process the effect of
chromatographic solvent demixing can also be considerably reduced. After
the last secondary front has left the sorbent layer and passed out through

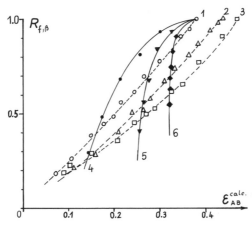

Fig. 5. Relationship between calculated eluent strength and R_f, β obtained using different apolar-polar mixtures on silica gel 60 (activated at 125°C for 30 min), temperature 30°C. 1, hexane-ethyl acetate; 2, hexane-THF; 3, hexane-acetone; 4, carbon tetrachloride-ethyl acetate; 5, benzene-ethyl acetate; 6, methylenechloride-ethyl acetate.

the outlet, the composition of the eluent becomes roughly constant, but equilibrium is still not achieved[11,12].

The last part of the development is achieved when the system attains perfect equilibrium. To make reproducible separations samples should only be injected in this period (as in HPLC). Up until this point the sorbent activity may change, except when isohydric solvents are used which are suited to the sorbent activity. In all other cases the changing water content of the eluent and sorbent result in different retentions in both the full off-line and full on-line OPLC systems.

If the water content of the sorbent bed was reduced by activation and the eluents used contain traces of water there is a good correlation between off-line and on-line retention as shown in Figure 3.

In the case of the xanthine separation using full off-line OPLC the dye Butter yellow moved with the secondary front. To convert this data to the on-line system the role of R_M additivity can be used: $^W R_{M,2} = R_{M,\beta} + R_{M,2}$, where $^W R_{M,2}$ is the R_M value in wet system, $R_{M,\beta}$ is the R_M value of the β-secondary front and $R_{M,2}$ is the R_M value of Butter yellow in the α-zone.

The full off-line and a partial on-line OPLC analytical separation of poppy alkaloids is shown in Figure 4. In this case the partial on-line OPLC system used involved off-line sample application, a prewetting from the outlet side and on-line separation/detection. As can be seen the retention of the components are in the same range.

The "PRISMA" model[16] is applicable to OPLC for selecting the eluents, but it is necessary to know that a multi-component apolar-polar solvent mixture will result in the formation of secondary solvent fronts.

In order to determine how the R_f's of the secondary (β) fronts depend on the eluent composition we measured the R_f values of β-front using different binary solvent systems. From this it was found that the $R_{f,\beta}$ versus logarithmic mole fractions of the polar component used in the mix-

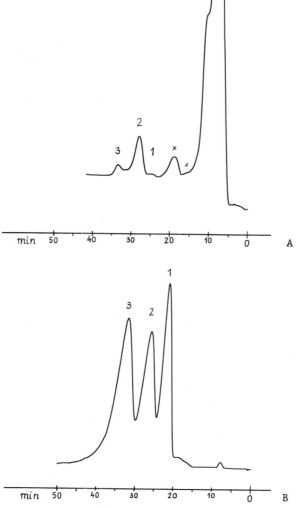

Fig. 6.   Full on-line separation of xanthines on preparative silica layer
with concentrating zone. External pressure on membrane, 2.5, MPa;
eluent, chloroform-acetic acid 60:40 v/v, 0.84 cm^3/min. 1,
theophylline; 3, theobromine; 2, caffeine. A - 1000 μl standard
solution, 3.2 mg/ml each; detection at 300 nm, AUFS 1; B - 1000
μl tea extract; detection at 300 nm, AUFS 0.5.

ture did not show a linear relationship. The eluent strength was calculated according to Snyder[17] and it was correlated with $R_{f,\beta}$ values
(Figure 5). At constant eluent strength the R_f β can be increased in such
a way as to eliminate the disturbances resulting from the demixing phenomena if the differences between the solvent strength of the components of
the solvent are kept as small as possible.

The last example described here concerns the use of OPLC for preparative isolation purposes. Thus Figure 6 shows the preparative full on-line
separation of xanthine standards (A) and a tea extract (B). It can be seen
that on-line OPLC is suitable for the efficient preparative separation of
natural products of this type with a loading of 0.54 x 10^{-4} g/g of sorbent
(K' = 2.47).

CONCLUSIONS

On-line and off-line OPLC have been shown to be useful planar chromatographic techniques suitable for both analytical and preparative scale separations. With careful choice of the solvent strength and of the components used in eluent mixtures disturbances due to solvent demixing can be reduced or eliminated.

REFERENCES

1. E. Tyihák and G. Held, in: "Progress In TLC And Related Methods," Vol. II, A. Niederwieser and G. Pataki, ed., Ann Arbor sci. Publ., Ann Arbor, Mich., (1971).
2. E. Tyihák, E. Mincsovics and H. Kalász, J.Chromatogr., 174:75 (1979).
3. E. Mincsovics, E. Tyihák, and H. Kalász, J.Chromatogr., 191:293 (1980).
4. H. Kalász, J. Nagy, E. Tyihák, and E. Mincsovics, J.Liquid Chromatogr., 3:845 (1980).
5. E. Tyihák, E. Mincsovics and F. Körmendi, Hung.Sci.Instru., 55:33 (1983).
6. E. Tyihák, T. J. Székely, and E. Mincsovics, in: Proc.2nd.Int.Symp.on Instrumental HPTLC, R. E. Kaiser, ed., Interlaken, Inst. for Chromatography, Bad Dürkheim, 159 (1982).
7. E. Tyihák and E. Mincsovics, in: Proc 3rd. Int. Symp. On Instrumental HPTLC, R. E. Kaiser, ed., Würzburg, p. 442 (1985).
8. E. Tyihák, E. Mincsovics, H. Kalász, and J. Nagy, J.Chromatogr., 211:45 (1981).
9. H. F. Hauck and W. Jost, J. Chromatogr., 262:113 (1983).
10. Zs. Fatér and E. Mincsovics, J.Chromatogr., 298:534 (1984).
11. E. Mincsovics, E. Tyihák and A. M. Siouffi, in: Proc.Int.Symp.TLC with Special Emphasis on OPLC, E. Tyihák, ed., Szeged (1984), Labor MIM Company, Budapest, p. 251.
12. L. R. Snyder and J. J. Kirkland, Introduction to Modern Liquid Chromatography (2nd. Ed.), J. Wiley and Sons Inc., New York (1979).
13. G. Guiochon, J.Chromatogr., 185:3 (1979).
14. N. Mellor, Chromatographia, 16:359 (1982).
15. A. Niederwieser and M. Brenner, Experientia, 21:50 (1965).
16. K. Dallenbach-Toelke, Sz. Nyiredy, B. Meier and O. Sticher, J. Chromatogr., 365:63 (1986).
17. L. R. Snyder, Principles of Adsorption Chromatography, Marcel Dekker, New York, Ch. 8. (1986).

ANTICIRCULAR PLANAR CHROMATOGRAPHY; ANALYTICAL

AND PREPARATIVE ASPECTS

H. Traitler and A. Studer

Nestlé Research Centre, Nestec Ltd
Vers-chez-les-Blanc
CH-1000 Lausanne 26, Switzerland

SUMMARY

The use of anticircular thin-layer (or planar chromatography) for analytical as well as preparative purposes, in particular in lipid chemistry, is described.

In addition anticircular TLC was compared with the linear technique and spot broadening was evaluated, calculated and expressed as a broadening factor. It could be shown that in both analytical and preparative anticircular TLC spot broadening was less pronounced than in comparable linear runs.

Typical analytical applications of anticircular planar chromatography were the separation and quantification of 5-hydroxytryptamides and tryptamines in food-products (including an on-plate derivatisation for detection) as well as unsaponifiable matters of plant lipids such as sterols, tocopherols, squalene and triterpenes. Fatty acids were also separated in preparative mode in order to obtain pure fractions for further identification using GC and GC/MS.

The preparative anticircular device was constructed for two particular reasons. Firstly in order to evaluate the performance of such a system, compared to a small anticircular separation U-chamber, and secondly to allow it to be tested in micropreparative separations.

INTRODUCTION

Anticircular planar chromatography as was developed by Kaiser represents a technique of thin-layer chromatography (TLC) involving several particular features such as annular sample deposition on the plate periphery, application of up to 24 samples per plate, absence of a chamber with consequently no chamber saturation necessary and, due to the fact of concentric migration, less spot broadening and diffusion than is usual in linear development.

Spot broadening, expressed as peak broadening, was compared for anticircular and linear techniques, respectively[1]. It can be expressed as the peak broadening index (RP), and calculated by the equation:

$$PB \quad = \quad PW \quad 1/2 \quad R_f \qquad\qquad (1)$$

where PW 1/2 is the peak width at half height and R_f the retention factor. PW 1/2 correlates positively with the chartspeed of the chromatographic printer but is negatively proportional to the scan speed of a TLC-scanner. Thus equation [1] has to be formulated:

$$PB \quad = \quad \frac{PW\ 1/2\ x\ SS}{R\ x\ CS} \qquad\qquad (2)$$

where SS is the scan speed in mm/s and CS the chart speed in cm/min.

Lower PB values, between 0.1 and 1, generally indicate little spot broadening (or diffusion) and are typical for anticircular development, whereas values between 1 and 2 or higher indicate pronounced spot broadening and pronounced diffusion, and are typical of non-vapor controlled linear development. For example the PB values for triterpenes and sterols in linear development were 0.92 and 1.23 respectively whilst the equivalent values obtained for the same compounds in anticircular development were 0.55 and 0.90.

Moreover, migration of the solvent is faster than in linear mode. For the separation of not too complex mixtures, this method is one of the easiest and most reliable TLC-modes and is particularly well suited to repetitive routine analyses.

One of the drawbacks of this method is at least on small 10 x 10 nano-plates, the short migration distance, approximately 4 cm maximum, which physically limits the number of compounds which can theoretically be resolved on such a plate.

The main interest of our work lies in the analytical evaluation of specific components of food and cosmetic products. In the following, we will discuss some examples of typical applications of anticircular planar chromatography in this area.

APPLICATION OF ANTICIRCULAR PLANAR CHROMATOGRAPHY

Determination of 5-hydroxytryptamides and serotonin[2]

Serotonin, which is found in animal and vegetable tissues, commands biological interest as a biogenic amine[3]. Its systematic name is 3-(2-aminoethyl)-5-indolol; it is also known as 5-hydroxytryptamine, and has the formula:

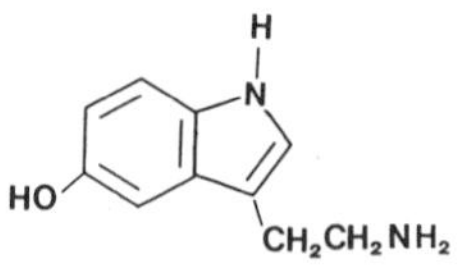

Fig. 1a.

The compound is sensitive to heat, light, and oxygen. Neither the chemical nature nor the biological activities of the reaction products are known so far. Several other phenolic compounds resembling serotonin occur in coffee wax but are present in smaller quantities.

68

The carboxylic acid of 5-hydroxytryptmine, isolated from coffee wax and other vegetable tissues (e.g. cocoa shells)[4], has the following structure[5]:

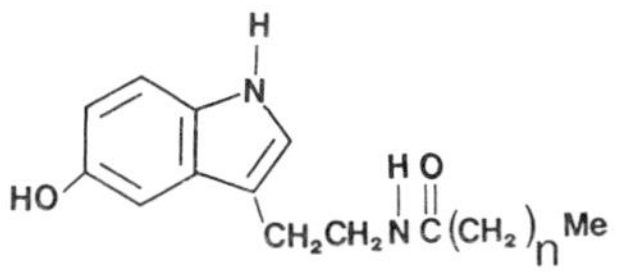

Fig. 1b.

Structural analyses have indicated the presence of three compounds derived from a combination of the primary amino group of 5-hydroxytryptamine and arachidic acid (n=18), behenic acid (n=20), or lignoceric acid (n=22) in a ratio of 12:12:1, respectively. In our shorthand notation, these compounds are called C-5-HT, and are only present in the surface wax of the bean.

Chromatography

In the present work anticircular HPTLC was applied to the particular separation problem. The apparatus used was a Camag "Anticircular U-Chamber". This simple method separates the previously extracted tryptamide component by migration of substances from the periphery to the center of the plate. The separation is fast, easily performed, and up to 24 samples could be analyzed on one plate. The standard was spotted with disposable micropipettes in quantities of 1 to 10µl of a 0.006% standard solution. The concentrations of the samples was chosen according to their C-5HT contents. Toluene/ethyl acetete (4:3) was used as mobile phase and the separation was terminated after 3-4 min. Then the plates were dried at ambient temperature for ca. 10 min. Subsequently the spots were visualized by the "dip-in" technique with Gibbs reagent for phenolic compounds (0.1% of 2,6-dichloroquinone-4-chlorimide in petroleum ether). The plate is usually fully developed after ca. 30 min. to produce light to dark blue spots according to the concentrations of samples. These spots were then fixed by spraying with 5% aqueous ammonia in methanol, and after another 30 min, scanning with visible light (540 nm) was performed. A Camag UV/VIS scanner was used for all measurements. This wavelength corresponded almost to the maximum absorption of the colored spot. This measurement should not be done later than 4 h after spraying with aqueous ammonia in order to avoid unreliable results due to degradation ("browning effect") of the plate.

On-plate Derivatization of Serotonin

Owing to the presence of a free amino group, serotonin does not react with Gibbs reagent to give a blue color. However, derivatisation of serotonin to an amide can be performed directly on the plate by over spotting the sample with a 5% solution of benzoyl chloride in toluene. It was found that 3 to 5 µl applications of this solution gave the best results. After drying, during which time the reaction goes to completion, analysis can be continued as described above. The intensity of visualized spots depends almost exclusively on substance concentration and not on the amount of reagent. Obviously, no such derivatization is necessary for 5-hydroxytryptamide.

The calibration curves for serotonin (as benzoylamide) and 5-hydroxy-tryptamide are shown in Figure 2. Practicable measuring ranges for both substances are between 1 and 10 µl spotted solutions corresponding to 0.115 µg/µl serotonin and 0.065 µg/µl tryptamide, respectively.

The determination and quantification of 5-hydroxytryptamine in cocoa shells and in cocoa powders possibly containing impurities of different amounts of shells is described as a practical example. It is known that cocoa beans themselves contain practically no tryptamide, whereas the amount of tryptamine in shells is about 75 ppm according to the present method. The correlation of the amount of tryptamide found with the composition of mixtures of various amounts of cocoa beans and shells is shown in Figure 3. The blank value of tryptamide for beans is up to ca. 2 ppm.

Four different commercial cocoa powders were analyzed with regard to possible determination and quantification of cocoa shell impurities. Two powders were found to contain practically no shell impurities (Cailler powder, 1.4 ppm; a Dutch powder, 2,1 ppm) and two powders contained amounts of tryptamide indicating small amounts of shell impurities (English powder 6.1 ppm corresponding to ca. 5% shells; a Swiss powder with 4.3 ppm corresponding to ca. 3% shell impurities).

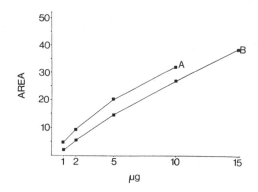

Fig. 2.   Calibration curves for serotonin (on-plate derivatized; 1 µl –
          0.115 µg) and hydroxytryptamide (1 µl – 0.065 µg).

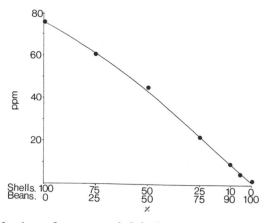

Fig. 3.   Correlation of amount of 5-hydroxytryptamide found with the
          composition of mixtures of cocoa shells and cocoa beans.

70

Determination of Lipids in Cosmetic Products

Another example is the direct determination of lipid compounds in cosmetic products.

In particular, we looked into the quantitative determination of jojoba wax - a long chain liquid wax ester - and shea butter fat, a tropical or so called wild fat.

The task here was to develop a simple, straightforward procedure to enable the analytical control of the fat components directly in the product avoiding lengthy extraction or clean-up procedures.

Jojoba Determination[6]

The cosmetic products were dissolved in a mixture of 75% dichloromethane and 25% methanol. The concentrations of the solutions were as follows: for a cream containing 4% jojoba wax, 0.5%, 0.25%, 0.1%, and 0.05%, and for a milk containing 1% jojoba wax, 2.0%, 1.0%, 0.4%, 0.2%, and 0.1%. The solutions obtained were transparent with practically no undissolved material.

Standards containing pure jojoba wax were prepared according to the jojoba content of the corresponding samples. The appropriate jojoba standard concentrations were: 0.02%, 0.01%, 0.004%, and 0.002% (w/v).

Fat Determinations

Under the given conditions, the total amount of glyceride fats could be determined at the same time. In this case, shea fat was used as the standard and the concentrations used were: 0.015%, 0.0075%, 0.003%, and 0.0015% (w/v).

Separation and Detection of Jojoba Wax and Total Glyceride Lipids

a) HPTLC separation. The anticircular U-chamber was used for this particular separation. The plate was washed twice with methanol, dried at 80°C, and cooled to ambient temperature.

After cleaning, a concentric ring of 7 mm diameter was scraped off in the middle to ensure more homogenous migration to the center of the plate. The samples were applied using a Nanomat spotter (Camag, Basel); 1.0 μl of each sample was spotted. The 10 x 10cm HPTLC plates (silica gel 60F$_{254}$, Merck, Darmstadt) were used to spot 12 to 24 samples. The separations were carried out with a mixture of petroleum ether (40°C dist.) and diethyl ether (60/40). Migration was completed after 3 min and the plate left to cool to about 25°C. For visualization, the plate was rapidly dipped into a 2% solution of phosphomolybdic acid/isopropanol and methanol (70:30 v/v). This reagent should not be more than 10 days old and must be stored in the dark. The plate was then dried with hot air for 2 min and heated in an oven at 120°C for 3 min.

b) Detection. The measurements, which had to be performed between 15 min and 2 h after visualization, were carried out using a UV-VIS scanner (Model No. 1, Camag, Basel) at 546nm. The spots were measured in the circular mode and the areas were recorded by a Spectra-Physics 4100 integrator.

The optimum concentration of spotted samples was in the range 0.02 to 0.1 µg/µl jojoba and 0.05 to 0.075 µg/µl shea fat (or other similar triglycerides), respectively. Sample concentrations have to be chosen accordingly. The method allows a wide range of jojoba or fat concentrations in cosmetic cream or milk to be measured. The solutions have to be adjusted according to the detection range.

Preparative Separation of Fatty Acids[7]

Another topic of interest for us is the separation of fatty acids or fatty acid methyl esters (FAMES) for subsequent structure elucidation with Ci GC-MS. One particular problem was to determine and confirm the double bond position of two fatty acids in the oil of the seeds of blackcurrants. We had identified them by multidimensional capillary gas chromatography as γ-linolenic acid (a metabolite of linoleic acid) and stearidonic acid, C18:4, n-3 (a metabolite of α-linolenic acid), peaks 6 and 8 of Figure 4.

As methyl esters, these compounds can be sufficiently well separated and create no resolution problem in direct GC/MS mode.

However, for the determination of the double bond locations, they had first to be converted into the corresponding pyrrolidides. Unfortunately, in this case linoleic and γ-linolenic acid elute very close to each other as is the case for α-linolenic and stearidonic acid. Planar chromatography on reversed phase plate material enabled us to separate linoleic from γ-linolenic and α-linolenic from stearidonic acid, respectively.

The different zones were scraped off, eluted and converted into the corresponding pyrrolidides[8]. This yielded unequivocal and readily interpretable mass spectra. Pyrrolidides of unsaturated fatty acids give stable intermediary fragments in electron impact MS and allow a "count-down" of the double bonds.

According to the general rule, fragment intervals of 12 mass units, which occur between the most intensive peaks of clusters of fragments

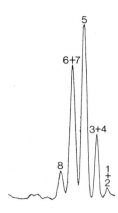

Fig. 4. HPTLC densitogram of black currant oil FAMES. Conditions: Nanoplate RP 18 (Merck) with solvents methanol/acetonitrile 1:1 dipping into 5% phosphomolybdic acid in acetone, charring at 150°C, 5 min. Scanning: Camag scanner, 546 nm, scanning speed 0.5 mm/sec. slit width 5 mm. Integration: Spectra Physics 4100, chart speed 4 cm/min, attenuation 128. (For peak numbers, see Table 1) Vertical figures indicate retention times as printed by the integrator.

Table 1.

Peak number	FAMES	% of total lipid FAME
1	C16:0	6-7
2	C18:0	1-2
3	C18:1 N-9 <u>cis</u>	9-10
4	C18:1 N-9 <u>trans</u>	0-5
5	C18:2 N-6 all <u>cis</u>	47-49
6	C18:3 N-6 all <u>cis</u> (γ-linolenic acid)	15-19
7	C18:3 N-3 all <u>cis</u>	12-14
8	C18:4 N-3 all <u>cis</u> (stearidonic acid)	3-4
U	unknown (from solvent)	

containing n and n-1 carbon atoms of the acid moiety, indicate the double bond as being located between carbons n and n + 1. Single bonds correspond to mass intervals of 14, whereas double bonds are indicated by mass intervals of 12 (9-11).

In this case, we were obliged to work in a micro-preparative way on an analytical anticircular U-chamber. This led us to the idea that by simply enlarging the system of the U-chamber, material deposition onto the plate

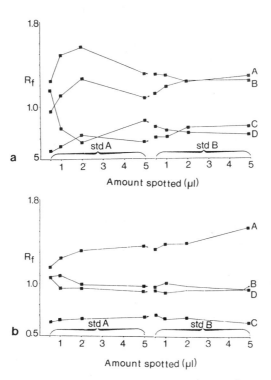

Fig. 5.   (a) Relation between concentration and response factors (on 10 x 10 cm plate).   Standard B = 10 times conc. A.   (b) Relation between concentration and response factor (on 20 x 20 cm plate). Standard B = 10 times conc. A.

could be increased and consequently we would have more substances available for subsequent analyses[1]. Thus we constructed a preparative anti-circular chromatography system (PACH) which works with 20 x 20 cm plate sizes. Migration time in this case is ca. 12 min (compared to some 3.5 min for the analytical U-chamber. To evaluate the performance of such a system, we compared the response linearity of the two anticircular devices, i.e. the analytical versus the preparative system.

The standard mixtures which we evaluated contained so-called lipid unsaponifiables, typically tocopherols, sterols, triterpenes and hydro-carbons.

It clearly can be seen that in the case of 20 x 20cm plates we obtain a better linearity at already low sample concentrations, whereas at higher concentrations this difference in performance can no longer be observed. (Figure 5).

CONCLUSION

Anticircular planar chromatography in its analytical as well as in its preparative form, represents a fast, reliable and highly reproducible exact method for the determination, quantitative evaluation and preparative separation of not too complex mixtures in particular in the field of food analysis.

This method is particularly useful for routine analyses involving a large number of samples and standard measurements.

REFERENCES

1. A. Studer and H. Traitler, J.High Resolut.Chromatogr.Chromatogr. Commun., 9:218 (1986).
2. A. Studer and H. Traitler, J. High Resolut.Chromatogr.Chromatogr. Commun., 5:581 (1982).
3. C. Garcia-Moreno, Alimentaria 93:21 (1978).
4. U. Harms, Dissertation, Hamburg (1986).
5. U. Harms and J. Wurziger, Z. Lebensmittelunters.Forsch. 138:75-80 (1968).
6. A. Studer and H. Traitler, J. High Resolut.Chromatogr.Chromatogr. Commun. 8:19 (1985).
7. H. Traitler, H. WInter, U. Richli and Y. Ingenbleek, Lipids 19:923 (1984).
8. W. Vetter, W. Walther and M. Vecchi, Helv.Chim.Acta., 54:1599 (1971).
9. B. A. Andersson and R. T. Holman, Lipids 9:185 (1974).
10. B. A. Andersson, W. W. Christie and R. T. Holman, Lipids 10:215 (1975).
11. T. Takagi and Y. Itabashi, Lipids 17:716 (1982).

RADIO-THIN-LAYER CHROMATOGRAPHY:

INSTRUMENTS AND APPLICATIONS

THE AMBIS TWO DIMENSIONAL BETA SCANNER

Ivor Smith

School of Pathology
Middlesex Hospital Medical School
London WIP 7LD

SUMMARY

The AMBIS two dimensional scanner will scan quantitatively any two dimensional surface such as thin-layer chromatography plates, gel electrophoresis, blot or whole body sections - for beta particle emission. The raw counts data of every spot or band can be printed out as total or percentage total radioactivity. A large range of software programs allows the comparison of any of the areas of interest stored in the memory, the determination of protein molecular weights, the production of taxonomic data bases, counting of dot blots, examination of whole body frozen sections, etc. Direct photography of the scan picture on the video monitor yields a picture practically identical to, and with the resolution of, an autoradiograph.

INTRODUCTION

Although a number of workers had experimented with the topic, the first practical, operational spark chambers were described by Pullan et al.,[1-2] in 1965 and their applications in chromatography by Hesselbo[3]. The original chambers were two dimensional and based on a set of anode wires with a further set of cathode wires running at right angles. Manufacture of such apparatus was fraught with difficulties as the wires tended to sag and short out. Later apparatus used coiled wire cathodes through which ran single anode wires resulting in a more stable arrangement. An apparatus based on Pullan's design was first manufactured in the early 1960's[3]. Beta particles emitted by the sample caused a spark discharge between the electrodes, hence the name spark chamber, and this spark was photographed on Polaroid film. Very satisfactory, qualitative, pictures were obtained. In the intervening two decades, advances in physics and computers have enabled methods for quantification to be developed together with a range of programs for manipulating the raw counts data.

The AMBIS beta scanner, based on a new design by Dr. Brian Pullan, is uniquely different from all other scanners in that it is a two dimensional scanner. All other scanners are one dimensional and based on a multiplicity of closely spaced, parallel wire anodes about 1cm long which limits the scan dimension to approximately that width. Any extension of the 1cm length makes this design inherently unstable as the longer wires tend to sag and touch and thus result in a diminished resolution. Hence such apparatus can only produce a two dimensional scan by building up repeated, adjacent one dimensional scans. The beta scanner is based on an entirely different approach with the result that the apparatus is much more stable and robust, as shown below.

Many experiments are short term and often completed within a few hours yet the subsequent autoradiography may take days, weeks or even months. Furthermore, the resulting autoradiograph (ARG) is often found to be under or over exposed, needs to be done again for a different time, and is usually only qualitative. For these reasons the ultimate design aim for the AMBIS was to produce, on screen, the equivalent of an ARG in minutes or hours and, by accumulating the data in a memory store, allow its manipulation in a variety of ways as described below.

All beta emitters, except tritium, many gamma emitters which emit secondary beta particles and alpha emitters can be detected and measured by the AMBIS scanner. By dropping the scan voltage, alpha particles can be detected whilst the beta and gamma emitters are not. Excellent results have been obtained with C14, S35, P32, Fe59, I125 and I131. Indeed, a number of pairs of primary and secondary beta emitters, such as I125 and I131, can be differentiated when present on the same gel.

The AMBIS Mk2 Beta Scanner

The AMBIS scanner was designed to be a two dimensional scanner and will scan the whole of any surface up to 20 x 20cm simultaneously. With the current computer, it is possible to display data from 274,176 points, that is points at approximately 0.4mm intervals on the scanned object. The surface may be a one dimensional (1D) or two dimensional (2D) TLC plate or electrophoresis gel or blot or even a whole body frozen section. Highly radioactive samples can be scanned in as short a time as 10-15 minutes although scans as long as 80 hr are possible. An accumulation facility allows the whole to be rescanned and added to the first set of scan data already in store. Hence if one had chosen a scan time which turned out to be insufficient, the add on facility ensures that the time was not wasted. As the accumulation of scanning data is a discrete operation, the computer plus software can be used simultaneously for other work such as the analysis of data held in the memory.

The principle on which the AMBIS Mk2 scanning head is based has been described in detail elsewhere[4] and so will be referred to only briefly here. From the top of the head down, there are a limited number of cathode strips with a similar small number of anode wires running beneath at right angles and separated by walls to reduce 'crosstalk'; these form a sturdy array of discrete, well-separated, proportional wire counters each seeing a small element of the sample. Then follows an aperture plate, a Mylar film to prevent ingress of radioactive particles and finally a resolution plate containing 28 holes in the X and 34 holes in the Y direction allowing the equivalent of 52 detector points. The sample plate or gel is pressed up to the head which scans these points. It is then lowered, moved, raised again and a second lot of adjacent points is scanned. In all the plate moves nine times in the X for each of eight times in the Y direction ultimately yielding a total of 72 x 52 = 8544 sets of counts which are integrated to form the completed scan data.

The major features of the MK2 scanning head are improved sensitivity and stability, better uniformity of response and lower background. This has resulted from a radically different mechanical and electrical design. The improvement in sensitivity is most marked for weakly ionising beta particles such as those from phosphorus 32. The new detector allows longer particle tracks within the detector gas without loss of spatial resolution, and also a much larger effective detector area. This larger detector area, or better area utilisation, results in a very significant increase in sensitivity when scanning at low spatial resolution. The new design also allows greater mechanical accuracy to be achieved in the construction of the detector and this, together with the improved sensitivity, leads to marked improvement in the uniformity of response. An important factor in determining the detectability of weak spots or bands is the background. The background of the new detector has been significantly reduced, both by the careful selection of materials and the use of an anti-coincidence guard or shield detector. Marked stability improvements result from the new design of amplification and data coding circuitry. Various other background removal and manipulation programs are provided. As background can be due to radioactive decomposition of the sample during the run and may result in unwanted counts over the 1D length or 2D area of the sample, an adjustable background allows this also to be removed. On first setting up the scanner and before scanning the first sample a 16 or 24 hr background without sample can be run and put into the memory. This set of counts is then used to compensate for extraneous counts due to cosmic rays and apparatus effects; the actual count is automatically adjusted to the subsequent scan time of each sample before subtraction from the sample data. However, as background can also be due to sample smearing, decomposition, etc. further variable and operator adjusted background can also be removed.

Resolution plates with different geometries are available and, for example, rectangular holes 3mm x 1.0 or 0.4mm are most suitable for scanning narrow bands whereas a 2 x 2mm hole is better for TLC or 2D spots. Scanner head support posts allow a variable height between the sample lifter plate and the underside of the resolution plate of up to 1.8cm so that thick samples such as microtitre plates can be scanned. With gels, a sensitivity of at least 50 dpm/2mm^2 spot in 60 minutes is found.

The system is controlled by an IBM PC AT computer using a high resolution monitor which allows the display of pictures practically identical with that seen on ARG's (see Figure 3). All menus are presented as single lines at the bottom of the screen and require only a single letter command. Thus the main menus is - S(can), P(rocess), A(nalyse), C(ompare). Pressing any one of these capitals brings up the appropriate subsidiary menu and some examples of each are shown. The Scan submenu shows (B)egin, (C)heck status, (R)etrieve, (E)xtend scan time, and (X)abort. The (P)rocess submenu places on the main area of the monitor a picture of the scan with, below, an indication of the centre of the lanes of a 1D and, at the side, a data summary including total counts, scan time, etc. (see Figure 1). Any area may then be enclosed in a box with adjustable X and Y coordinates when the data in the defined area or lane can be extracted and separately stored in the memory (see Figures 1 and 3). Simultaneously a histogram of the lane appears on the side at the left. The A(nalyze) submenu allows lanes previously extracted to be quantified in total, bands and spots to be marked and individually quantified, molecular weights of proteins in gels to be determined, etc. Where the activities in the different lanes or areas vary appreciably, they can be completely or partially scaled up or down over a very wide range so that even the weakest of lanes or spots can be brought up for comparison with other lanes or spots which may even have to be scaled down (see Figures 5 and 7). Similarly, spots and areas on 2D and even whole body scans can be boxed and quantified. C(ompare) allows any lane to be compared with any other lane in the memory (see Figure 3) and, to ensure good matching, any lane or part of a lane may be normalised by lengthwise stretching or compressing to improve fit. Finally, every screen picture can be printed out although actual screen images are best photographed as they are then ready for publication.

APPLICATIONS

Thin-Layer Chromatography

The simplest operations to perform are those applicable to 1D and 2D
TLC because all that is required is the basic scan operation followed by
quantitation of the spots. An interesting example of such an application
is shown in Figure 1. It shows the TLC of an enzyme assay of importance in
transfection experiments. Chloramphenicol is incubated with 14C-acetyl CoA
to determine the presence of the enzyme, acetyltransferase, and then the
mixture is run by TLC to separate the acetylchloramphenicol formed. Each
lane is the result of one experiment and boxing of the lane followed by
quantitation gives a measure of the enzyme present. The 2D TLC of a single
pure drug which decomposes during the chromatographic run is illustrated in
Figure 2. The sample was applied at the bottom right hand corner and run
(shown horizontally in the figure). The plate was turned and run in the
same solvent after the application of a further spot of the drug at the
right. The major spot, some 72% of the total radioactivity, can be seen to
decompose into a number of products, some of which appear to be stable and
some unstable when run in the second direction; the major spot also decomposes further in the second run. Every spot has been quantified but the
data are not reported here.

Gel Electrophoresis

Scanning is particularly valuable after gel electrophoresis of radiolabelled proteins. Whole micro-organisms, animal cells or sub-cellular
fractions can be labeled with S35-methionine or S35-thioATP or a range of
other radioactive compounds. The macromolecules are released into solu-

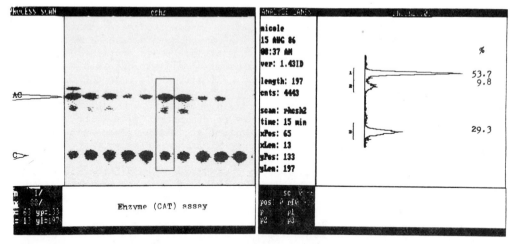

Fig. 1. Quantitative enzyme assay by TLC. Chloramphenicol (C) was
         incubated with [14C-acetyl]CoA in the presence of chlor-
         amphenicol-acetyltransferase when acetylchloramphenicol (AC) was
         formed. Ten samples were incubated, chromatographed on a TLC
         plate, scanned for 15 min. and one lane enclosed in a box as shown
         in the left of the figure. The boxed lane was extracted, and the
         (A)nalyse menu used to place a histogram on screen as shown in the
         right hand figure. The peaks are marked, using the arrow seen at
         the base of the lowest peak, and quantified. A print out for any
         or all peaks was then obtained by pressing the P button although
         the actual figures have been added at the side of the peaks for
         this figure in order to save space.

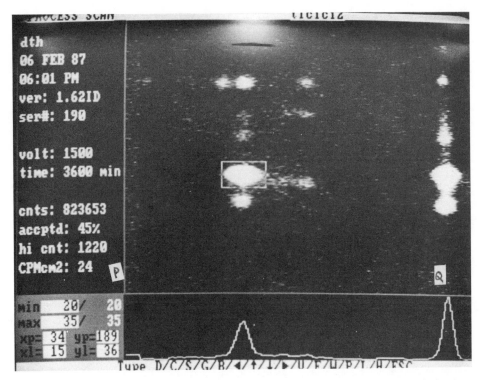

Fig. 2. Two dimensional TLC of a pure drug. This drug decomposed during chromatography. It was applied at point P and chromatographed in a solvent in the horizontal direction of the figure. After drying, the plate was turned at right angles, a second spot of the drug applied at point Q and chromatographed in the same solvent. The drug has been boxed and quantified at 72%, after the second run. It is interesting to try and determine which substances derived from the first decomposition are stable in the second run. This was a 60 h scan.

tion, treated with SDS and mercaptoethanol, and electrophoresed by standard methods.

Figure 3 shows an acrylamide gel separation of 15 samples which was scanned for 60 minutes. The video screen is photographed directly and appears practically identical with that found on an ARG requiring some days or even longer. Lane 11 has been enclosed by a box whose X and Y dimensions have been adjusted to enclose that part of the lane which is of interest and this has been "extracted" to produce the histogram on the left. A visual examination shows that this histogram corresponds with the band intensities. The submenu capital letters below allow one to D(isplay) any named scan image in the memory, alter the C(ontrast), S(ummarise) the data relating to the scan, draw a B(ox) around the lane, adjust the XY coordinates with the arrows, G(rid), E(xtract) the lane data into the memory, P(rint) and obtain H(elp) which explains all the letters. The data shown in the left hand bottom corner indicates the maximum and minimum counts per pixel, these being 1 and 354 but the maximum has been reduced to 140 indicating that every spot with counts of 140+ has been set at 140 for maximum intensity. The right-hand side of Figure 3 shows two extracted lanes taken from the memory and redrawn onto the screen for comparison purposes. Electrophoresis runs are not always identical for a number of

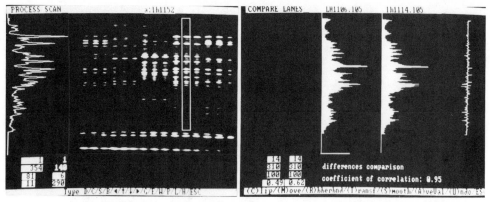

Fig. 3. Gel electrophoresis and comparison of two lanes. 15 samples were
run on the AMBIS electrophoresis unit (not discussed in this
chapter, but see reference 4), the gel was dried, scanned for 30
min and processed. The samples were set up in triplicate at
different concentrations. Lane 11 was boxed and its histogram
appears at the left. On the right, the same sample run on two
different gels is being examined in the (C)ompare mode. Both the
difference pattern, shown on the far right, and the coefficient of
correlation, printed out below, indicate identity of the sample in
the two lanes.

reasons. Hence it is possible to C(lip) off the top and or bottom of the
run, S(mooth) the raw histogram, R(ubberband), i.e. expand or contract the
lane, and U(ndo) an operation in order to get a best fit measure. The far
right shows a difference result after automatically subtracting the right
from left lane which yields evidence of identity and the coefficient of
correlation value concludes the identity analysis. The data in the left
corner indicate the lengths of the Y axis used, the fact that the counts
have been averaged to 100 and the amount of scaling down of each lane to
allow the best comparison.

Other valuable procedures for protein studies are the determination of
molecular weights, quantitation of particular bands and 2D scans. A composite figure from a number of screen printouts derived from a study of the
subdivision of strains of a mycobacterium (BCG) by uptake of S35-
methionine[5] - a standard procedure in microbiological taxonomy is shown
in Figure 4. Molecular weight standards (ST) run in parallel with the
radio-labelled proteins allow a molecular weight calibration curve to be
drawn via the appropriate software so that the MW's of any of the proteins
in other lanes on the gel can be readily determined. Over twenty such
protein bands in the sample can be marked and similarly calibrated. The
peaks can also be quantified as total counts and as a percentage of the
total counts in the lane.

Two dimensional electrophoresis runs can also be examined. On the
right of Figure 4 is a composite '2D' scan which is particularly easy to do
on the AMBIS 2D scanner. Two samples of the same BCG specimen are run on a
non-denaturing gel. The lanes are cut out of the first gel, one is placed
at the top of a second, denaturing gel and run in the second dimension with
MW standards. After the run, the other lane is aligned with the second gel
and the whole is scanned. Mathematical calculation of the MW of the major
spot in the first gel shows it to be 46K but it produces a single spot of
MW 23K in the second run. Hence it is a dimer containing two identical
subunits. Once the data is stored, it too can be screened over a wide

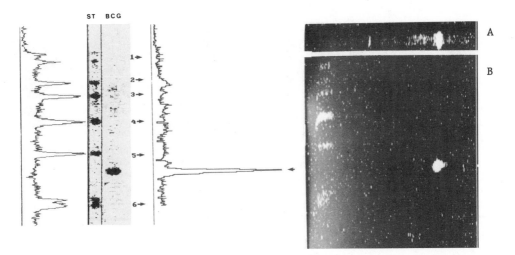

Fig. 4.   Molecular weight program.   This is a composite figure made up from
a number of screen figures.   A mycobacterium (BCG) was grown in
the presence of radioactive methionine.   The cells were removed
and the supernatent was treated with SDS-mercapteothanol.   A gel
was run with radioactive protein standards (ST) of known MW's in
parallel with the proteins secreted by the BCG, dried and scanned.
A histogram of the ST's in the (A)nalyse mode was screened (left)
and the MW's of each peak was read into the memory.   The BCG lane
was then screened, the pointer moved to the major peak, the Q key
pressed when the position of the six ST's and the calculated MW is
printed on screen; the MW is not shown here because of scale
differences in the photography.   (Taken from reference 5 with
permission).   On the right is the corresponding 2D run.   Two
samples were run in parallel lanes on the same non-denaturing gel.
One lane was cut off, placed at the top of an SDS denaturing gel
together with a drop of MW standards and run (gel B).   No well was
available in which to place the MW sample and this explains the
rather poor spots on the electrophoresis.   The second 1D gel (A)
was aligned with the 2D gel for scanning together.

range of sensitivities as shown in Figure 5.   Using a high background, only
slightly lower than the maximum spot count recorded, only the most radioactive spots appear.   Dropping the background, a much larger number of
spots appears and, with minimum background, even the most minor spots can
be observed.   Because the print out is a 1:1 scale, the positions of the
most radioactive spots can be determined and covered with thick foil so
that, on rescanning, minor spots in these areas can also be located.
Clearly this one scan can be made equivalent to a very large number of
ARG's exposed for a number of different times but at the cost of just a
single scan which is itself less expensive than one ARG.

Microbiology and Taxonomy

The operational software described above for stretching and compressing lanes obviously includes within it the facility for pattern recognition
and matching, and brings a new dimension to the investigation of problems
such as the identification and comparison of microorganisms in microbiology
and numerical taxonomy.   Most workers still rely on visual comparison
although a few have developed what must now be considered as rather slow
computer programs requiring a great deal of input and manipulation time.
The AMBIS system software, with its 30 Mbyte hard disc store, allows the

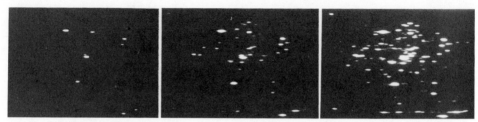

Fig. 5. Contrast alteration. This figure of a 2D electrophoresis gel
illustrates how widely the contrast can be altered. On the left
the background has been increased to just below that of the spots
with the highest count so that only the most radioactive spots
will be seen. As the background is reduced the next most active
spots are observed (middle) and then, with minimum background
(right), even the weakest spots can be observed.

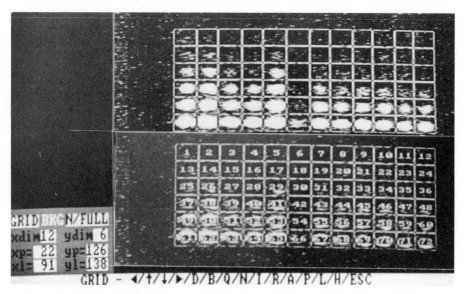

Fig. 6. Regular array spot quantification. Dot blots, or spots applied
from column or other fractions, were scanned and screened. A
variable grid was placed on and adjusted around the spots by
keying in the appropriate number of vertical and horizontal lines.
The boxes could be individually numbered as shown. When the
quantification key, with or without a suitable background, was
pressed the number of counts was printed in each box to two
figures (although the print out will give full counts to four
figures plus a statistical analysis). Data on any one box number
could be extracted separately.

continuous construction and update of a dynamic database, immediate comparison of a new organism pattern with the whole of the patterns in store,
an on screen selection of the pattern with the highest spectral match and
coefficient of correlation, a list of the next nine alternate matches with
correlation coefficients and a Z-score of peaks in the two lanes which fall
within selected standard deviations.

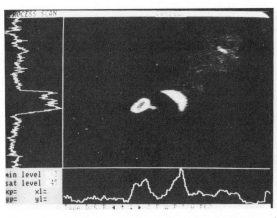 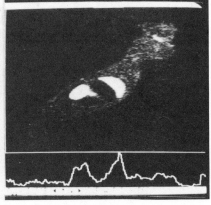

Fig. 7. Whole body scan. A radioactive drug was administered to a rat. After a suitable time the rat was rapidly frozen in liquid nitrogen and a microtome frozen section taken for scanning. The left hand scan at high background shows that the majority of the drug is concentrated in the liver and kidney with a little taken up in the pituitary and other parts of the head. Note that the drug was concentrated in the kidney cortex and that the medulla is free of activity. With a much lower background the kidney uptake is blurred but the whole body outline can be observed together with the disposition of minor quantities of drug in the head and neck area. Because of the 1:1 printout, radioactive spots can be located and removed for TLC to determine whether the original drug or its metabolites are present in any area.

Blots and Spots

Dot blots, column fractions applied as spots, microtitre well extracts, ext can be scanned and counted using a simple grid program. An example whereby an XY grid can be set up to encompass the evenly placed spots simply by reading in the number of lines required on each axis is shown in Figure 6. Above is the actual scan of the dots enclosed in the grid. Below is a display of the numbering of the boxes. Counts of each sample can then be placed in each box to two significant figures. The factor by which the numbers must be multiplied for the correct scale of counts and other data can be placed on screen if desired. Of course, the print out provides the exact numbers to four figures together with CPM and percent of total grid activity.

Whole Body Frozen Sections

A quite different application is that of scanning whole body dried frozen sections. A scan of a rat section is shown in Figure after administration of a radioactive drug. Here the drug is clearly localised in the liver and kidney with minor amounts in the brain area. Examination at high background subtraction shows that the drug is sharply localised in the kidney cortex and nothing is in the medulla. This example, taken from an industrial application, is an extremely cost effective analysis as the result is obtained in a few hours instead of a few weeks.

ACKNOWLEDGEMENTS

The loan of an AMBIS system together with software updates from the manufacturers, Automated Microbiology Systems, Grundy Building, Somerset Road, Teddington, Middlesex and Automated Microbiology Systems, Inc., San Diego, California is acknowledged.

REFERENCES

1. B. R. Pullen and B. J. Perry, Ist. Int.Conf.on Medical Physics, Harrogate, England (1965).
2. B. R. Pullen, R. Howard, and B. J. Perry, Nucleonics 24:72 (1966).
3. T. Hesselbo, in: "Chromatographic and Electrophoretic Techniques," Ivor Smith (ed.), Vol. 1. Heinemann Medical Books, 2nd. ed. chp.27 p. 693, (1969).
4. Ivor Smith, BioEssays, 3:225 (1985).
5. C. Abou-Zeid, Ivor Smith, J. Grange, Jenny Steele and G. Rook, J.Gen.Microbiol., 132:3047 (1986).

THE ACCURACY AND REPRODUCIBILITY OF RADIO-THIN LAYER

CHROMATOGRAPHY MEASUREMENTS OF DRUGS IN BIOLOGICAL FLUIDS

F. A. A. Dallas, T. J. Halliday and D. A. Saynor

Glaxo Group Research Limited
Department of Biochemical Pharmacology
Priory Street, Ware, Herts, SG12 0DJ, UK

SUMMARY

The accuracy and reproducibility of radio-thin layer chromatography
(RTLC) of radiochemicals in biological fluids was investigated using a RITA
6800 analyzer. When applications were made in a simple matrix (water) with
no elution of the plate the accuracy of RTLC was comparable with liquid
scintillation counting (LSC). However at low loadings (92 dpm) the standard deviations were more than ten times greater with RTLC than LSC. With
spots of approximately 2mm in diameter the position of the detector wire
was not critical (± 3mm). Increasing concentrations of biological fluids
decreased the number of counts obtained. This was probably caused by a
change in the spatial distribution of the radiochemical in the silica.
Absorption of the radioactivity by constituents of the biological fluid was
not an important factor.

INTRODUCTION

For at least the last fifteen years this laboratory has been using
radio-thin layer chromatography (RTLC) in absorption, distribution, metabolism and excretion (ADME) studies. The technique has mainly been used for
obtaining metabolite profiles of drugs in biological fluids such as bile,
plasma and urine.

Analysis of the radioactivity on the TLC plate has been performed
using several methods[1] including:-

(a) Scraping the silica layer off the plate and analyzing the resulting
     powder by liquid scintillation counting (LSC).
(b) Autoradiography.
(c) Panax radio-scanner.
(d) Berthold radio-scanner[2].
(e) TLC analyzers such as the Berthold and Raytest RITA.

The earlier methods a-d all had major disadvantages either in that
they were time consuming, lacked sensitivity or were not easily used for
quantification. With the advent of the RTLC analyzers (e) however a whole
new area of applications became viable. The RTLC analyzers improved the
sensitivity and resolution of the detection system, reduced the analysis

time per sample dramatically and allowed quantification of chromatograms[3-5]. Most importantly all these attributes were to be found in the
one instrument.

The method that has been used is extremely simple. A known amount of
the biological fluid, and therefore a known amount of radioactivity, is
applied to the thin-layer chromatography (TLC) plate. The plate is eluted
with solvent, dried and the radioactivity present analyzed by a suitable
technique or detector. After analysis of the plate using the RTLC analyzer, the amounts of radioactivity in each region of interest (ROI) are
obtained and quoted as a percentage of the total radioactivity in all the
ROIs. From the amount of radioactivity in the sample, the concentration of
each component is calculated.

In our laboratory we only use the technique semi-quantitatively as,
although RTLC is widely used, we have been unable to find any information
on the accuracy and reproducibility of the technique.

The objective of these experiments was therefore to ascertain the
accuracy and reproducibility of the RTLC technique. We also wanted to
determine what factors, if any, affected the accuracy and reproducibility
and as a byproduct of the work to estimate the errors involved in the
various procedures used in the technique i.e. machine errors (background
and position) and application errors (volume and spatial distribution).

The factors that might affect the technique are numerous:

1) Non-linearity of response of the detector wire to varying amounts of
radioactivity. The response of the detector wire has been shown (J.
Clapham, personal communication) to be linear over a large range.

2) Non-linearity of response along the length of the detector wire. To
negate any effects of this type of non-linearity the instrument was set up
so that the response along the wire was as linear as possible. The application sites were also identical on each track and plate. Therefore, where
necessary, comparisons were always made on results obtained from the same
part of the detector wire.

3) Position (parallel displacement) of the detector wire. This would
only affect the technique if the chromatogram had not eluted perpendicularly to the origin, or if inter-track comparisons were to be made.

4) Spatial distribution of the radio-material within the silica. If the
distribution of radio-material within the silica varied from one spot to
the next then different degrees of absorption of the radioactivity by the
silica may occur. This might be the case when applications are made in
different biological fluids, if different elution systems were used, or if
poor chromatography resulted in variable Rf values.

5) Effects of the biological fluid. Different biological fluids or
variations in the constituents of any single biological fluid may affect
the technique indirectly by varying the spatial distribution of the radio-
material within the silica or directly by absorption of the radioactivity
to varying degrees.

Initially it was decided to investigate simple models which allowed
the determination and understanding of the effects of one or two of the
factors involved in the technique, whilst recognizing that the model itself
might bear little relation to the real technique. As more information was
obtained the complexity of the model was increased until finally the conditions were similar to those normally used.

The results obtained from these experiments also allowed a preliminary investigation of the errors in RTLC to be undertaken.

EXPERIMENTAL

Equipment and Chemicals

A RITA 68000 with version 2.0 software (Raytest Ltd., Sheffield) was used for the analyses. The analysis conditions were as follows:- voltage, 1615V; gas flow, 1.5 litres 10% methane in argon/min. saturated with methanol; preset time, 10 minutes; preset count, 20,000; discriminators, 60-200.

The quantity of radioactivity in each solution was determined by LSC with external standard channels ratio technique for quench correction. The LSC was performed in a Tracor Analytic Model 6882 Mark III liquid scintillation system (Denley Instruments Ltd.). Pico-Fluor 30 liquid scintillation cocktail was obtained from Packard Instrument Co.

UV (220nm) adsorption chromatograms were obtained using a Camag TLC II scanner obtained from Baird and Tatlock Ltd.

Microcaps (1µl) were obtained from the Drummond Scientific Co. and Merck silica gel 60 (0.25mm, F_{254}) TLC plates from BDH Chemicals Ltd. All solvents used were of Analar grade.

Radiochemicals

Four compounds (1 to 4, specific activity 50-200µCi/mg), each with one atom of carbon-14 were, obtained from the Isotope Laboratory, Chemical Development Department, Glaxo Group Research, Ware. Non-radiolabelled compound 1 was obtained from the same source.

Experimental Design

Each plate had a grid (6 x 6) of allowable application sites. These sites were 2.5, 5.5, 8.5, 11.5, 14.5 and 17.5cm from the edge of the plate in both the X and Y axis.

Each column of the grid was designated as a track (T1-T6) and each row of the grid was designated as a position (P1 - P6) however, in some experiments e.g. exp. 1, not all the available positions were used. Each track therefore consisted of six application sites (P1-P6) and was the equivalent of a lane on a normally developed plate.

ROIs were preset with a length of 20mm with the application site at the center.

Experiment 1: The Effect of Altering the Position of the Detector Wire

A track containing 6 spots of radioactivity (of 0, 92, 182, 633, 1802 and 7113 dpm respectively) was used for this experiment. Two separate analyses were performed.

a) The detector wire was offset at different distances (-3, -2, -1, 0, +1, +2, +3mm) from, but parallel to, the track. Four analyses were done at each position. The intra- and inter-track means and standard deviations of the total counts in all the ROIs were calculated.

b)   The detector wire was offset as before but by as much as 9mm (0 - +9mm
     at 1mm increments). Only one analysis at each position was performed.

Experiment 2: Accuracy and Reproducibility with water as the Matrix With no Elution of the TLC Plate

     Solutions of compound 1 (1mg/ml) containing 92 (A), 182 (B), 633 (C),
1802 (D) and 7113 (E) dpm were prepared. Portions of each solution were
analyzed by LSC. One application (1μl) of each solution was made to each
track (T2-T6) on each of four identical plates. Solution A was applied at
P2, solution B at P3, solution C at P4, solution D at P5 and solution E at
P6. P1 on each track was used as a background and T1 was not used. Each
track was analyzed four times. Intra- and inter-track means and standard
deviations of the counts within each ROI were calculated for each position
(P2-P6). For each track the counts within each ROI were also expressed as
a percentage of the total counts within all the ROIs. The means and standard deviations of the percentages were also calculated.

Experiment 3: Effect of Overspotting with biological Fluid

     A solution of compound 1 (1299dpm/μl) was applied (1μl) to P2-P6 in
T2-T6. P1 on each track was used as a background and T1 was not used.
Each track was analyzed four times. Three such plates were prepared and
analyzed.

     The same application sites (P2-P6) on one plate were then overspotted
(1μl) with varying dilutions of control dog bile in water (water, T2; 10%
bile, T3; 30% bile, T4; 70% bile, T5; 100% bile, T6). the plate was re-
analyzed as before.

     The other two plates were overspotted with similar dilutions of con-
trol dog plasma or urine and also re-analyzed.

     Intra-and inter-position and track means and standard deviations of
the counts were calculated for each plate before and after over-spotting
with biological fluid.

Experiment 4: Effect of Application in Biological Matrix

     Solutions of compound 1 were made up in varying dilutions of bio-
logical fluid (water, 10, 30, 70 and 98% biological fluid) such that 1μl of
each solution contained approximately 1745dpm. The solutions (1μl) were
applied to the TLC plate as in experiment 3. Three TLC plates were prepared (bile, plasma and urine). Tracks T2-T6 were each analyzed four
times. Means and standard deviations of the counts within the ROI's were
calculated as in experiment 3.

Experiment 5: Effect of Elution of Compound After Application in Biological Fluid

     A mixture (13960dpm/μl) containing compounds 1 to 4 in the ratio 16.5
: 16.5 : 57 : 10 respectively was prepared. This mixture was then mixed
with varying amounts of either bile, plasma or urine from 0 to 94% and
spotted onto the TLC plates.

     Applications (1μl) of each dilution (water, T2; 10%, T3; 30%, T4; 70%,
T5; 94%, T6) were made 2cm from the bottom edge of the tlc plate. Three
such plates (one each for bile, plasma and urine) were prepared.

The plates were then eluted for 10cm from the application site using dichloromethane-methanol-0.88 aqueous ammonia solution (80:10:1) as solvent.

Each track was analyzed four times. A portion of the TLC plate above the solvent front of each track was used as a background. Intra- and inter-track means and standard deviations of the counts in each ROI were calculated.

RESULTS

Experiment 1: Effect of position of the Detector Wire

The effect of offsetting the detector wire from the track is shown in Figure 1. When the detector wire was offset by up to 3mm on either side of the track no significant difference in the total counts was observed. Indeed an offset of greater than 3mm was required before any appreciable decrease in the number of counts detected was observed.

The standard deviations of the results were similar to the machine errors obtained when the detector wire was not offset (Table 5). This would be expected as all the analyses were of the same track and therefore no application error should be present.

The results suggest that for a small spot (the spot diameter was approximately 2mm) the position of the detector wire was not a critical factor with respect to the accuracy or reproducibility of the technique.

Experiment 2: Accuracy and Reproducibility with Water as Matrix and with No Elution of the TLC Plate

A comparison of the accuracy and reproducibility of the RTLC and LSC techniques is shown in Table 1.

As can be seen there was very little difference between the mean values obtained by RTLC as compared with LSC. In fact only one result was significantly different. However, the standard deviation of the RTLC technique was considerably larger (a factor > 10X) when only small amounts of radioactivity (92dpm) were applied to the TLC plate.

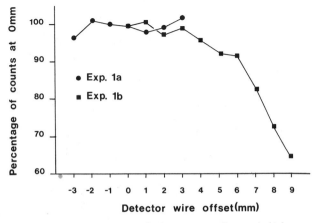

Fig. 1. Effect of detector wire position.

Table 1. Comparison of the Accuracy and Reproducibility of Radio-Thin Layer Chromatography (RTLC) and Liquid Scintillation Counting (LSC)

Position	Radioactivity applied (dpm)	% of Component ± SD (1)		% Difference (2)	$\dfrac{\text{SD RTLC}}{\text{SD LSC}}$
		RTLC	LSC		
P2	92	1.0000 ± 0.1866	0.9360 ± 0.0161	+ 6.8	11.6
P3	182	1.9956 ± 0.1897	1.8534 ± 0.0378	+ 7.7 (3)	5.0
P4	633	6.6000 ± 0.2798	6.4439 ± 0.0943	+ 2.4	3.0
P5	1802	18.0953 ± 0.4234	18.3470 ± 0.2362	− 1.4	1.8
P6	7113	72.3094 ± 0.5929	72.4198 ± 0.2166	− 0.2	2.7

(1) SD = standard deviation (n−1), n=80

(2) $\dfrac{\text{% RTLC} - \text{% LSC}}{\text{% LSC}}$ x 100

(3) ● Significant difference (p < 0.05)

Experiment 3: Effect of Overspotting with Biological Fluid

A comparison of the results obtained before and after overspotting with a biological fluid is shown in Table 2. These show that the counts detected decrease with increasing application of biological fluid.

As was expected there was also a slight decrease in the counts when the application sites were overspotted with water. The application of the water will alter the spatial distribution of the original spot and cause more of the radioactivity to be absorbed by the silica particles of the TLC plate. This result also indicated that the decrease in the counts obtained after overspotting with biological fluid may also be caused by a change in the spatial distribution of the radioactivity within the spot. However the proportion of the decrease that can be attributed to either a change in spatial distribution (absorption by the silica) or an absorption effect of the biological fluid cannot be obtained from this experiment.

Experiment 4: Effect on Counts of Application in Biological Fluid

A comparison of the counts obtained with different concentrations of biological fluids is shown in Table 3.

The results showed a similar, but accentuated, trend to that observed in Experiment 3. Thus counts decreased with increasing concentration of biological fluid. With both plasma and urine the decrease in the number of counts was much greater than in Experiment 3.

Again one cannot separate the effects of changes in the spatial distribution and absorption effects of the biological fluid. Suffice it to say that the biological fluid dramatically affected the number of counts obtained even when the TLC plate had not been eluted.

Experiment 5: Effect of Application in Biological Fluid and Elution

A chromatogram of the result obtained when the radioactive mixture applied in 70% bile was eluted with the solvent is shown in Figure 2. The chromatograms of the mixture applied in the other biological fluids were all very similar. The figure also shows a representative UV scan (220mm) of a biological fluid. Only three peaks were visible in the chromatogram because both compounds 1 and 2 have a similar Rf value in this solvent system. The first radioactive peak had a similar Rf to that of the major UV peak of the biological fluids and that the third radioactive peak had an Rf at which no UV peaks were found.

The proportion of the counts detected for each biological fluid as a percentage of the total counts in the 10% biological fluid sample is shown in Table 4. The results showed that for total counts there was a progressive decrease in the number obtained with increasing concentration of biological fluid. The results from the applications in water appeared to be different from any of the biological fluid results.

If the reduction in the number of counts were caused by quenching of the matrix we would have expected the counts in the first peak (where the UV peak is largest) to decrease to a greater extent than either of the other two peaks. However quite the reverse was true. There was very little decrease in the counts in peaks 1 and 2. Virtually all the decrease in the total counts was reflected in the decrease of the counts in peak 3. At this Rf there were no corresponding UV peaks at 220nm in any of the biological fluids.

Table 2. Effect on Counts of Overspotting with Biological Fluid

Matrix Concentration (%)	Total counts and % of counts (1)								
	Bile			Plasma			Urine		
	Before	After	%	Before	After	%	Before	After	%
Water	1639	1528	93	1679	1540	92	1632	1589	97
10	1749	1304	75	1676	1450	87	1695	1495	88
30	1768	1152	65	1766	1512	86	1691	1393	82
70	1772	976	55	1701	1293	76	1602	1251	78
100	1748	776	44	1701	1175	69	1644	1266	77

N = 20

(1) $\dfrac{\text{Counts after overspotting}}{\text{Counts before overspotting}}$ x 100

Table 3. Effect on Counts of Application in Biological Fluid

Counts and % of Counts in Water (1)

Matrix Concentration (%)	Bile		Plasma		Urine	
	Counts	%	Counts	%	Counts	%
Water	2107	100	1988	100	1941	100
10	1454	69	1737	87	1650	85
30	1043	50	1432	72	1619	83
70	978	46	1114	56	1287	66
98	1014	48	1110	56	1138	59

n = 20

(1) $\dfrac{\text{Counts in biological fluid}}{\text{Counts in water}}$ x 100

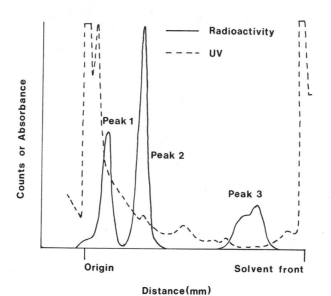

Fig. 2. Typical radioactivity and UV chromatogram of a mixture of radiochemicals in a biological fluid (bile).

These results together with those from Experiment 2 and 3 suggest that, although the biological fluid reduces the counts obtained, the effect must be a spatial distribution change causing increased absorption of the radioactivity by the silica and not by direct absorption of the radio-activity by the biological fluid.

Preliminary Investigation of the Errors Involved in RTLC

Variation in natural background, with position, with gas flow, with methanol saturation of gas, electronic noise and variations induced by changes in environmental conditions (e.g. atmosphere pressure) may all influence the final result and have all been classed in this investigation as machine error.

Variation in the volume applied and variation in the spatial distribution of the sample (which may again be caused by a variety of reasons) have been classed as application error.

In these experiments the errors are quoted as standard deviations (S). The machine error (S_M), the application error (S_A) and the total error (S_T) may be obtained from the experimental data or derived by using the formula,

$$S_T^2 = S_M^2 + S_A^2$$

Similar procedures have been used in the analysis of errors in TLC[5,6].

An estimation of the experimental and some derived errors is shown in Table 5. The results showed that all the errors increased with increasing amounts of radioactivity. However the increase in the machine error was much less than the increase in the application error.

When small amounts of radioactivity were applied the machine error was virtually equal to the total error. This was evident when the results of the error in the blank determination were compared. Obviously for the

Table 4. Effect on Counts of Application in Biological Fluid and Elution

| Matrix | % of Counts of 10% Biological Fluid | | | |
	Peak 1	Peak 2	Peak 3	Total
Water	84	97	59	82
10% Bile	100	100	100	100
30% "	96	98	99	98
70% "	102	102	73	93
94% "	96	98	60	86
Water	92	99	92	95
10% Plasma	100	100	100	100
30% "	97	98	92	96
70% "	94	94	91	93
94% "	90	94	81	89
Water	93	101	104	100
10% Urine	100	100	100	100
30% "	99	100	101	100
70% "	99	103	90	98
94% "	92	100	78	91

n = 4

blank no application of radioactivity was made therefore no application error should be present.

However when large amounts of radioactivity were applied the application error was much larger than the machine error and virtually equal to the total error.

The validity of deriving any one of the errors was also investigated. As we can see from Table 5 the experimental and calculated application errors were very similar.

DISCUSSION

Inherently, that is with no elution of the plate and a relatively simple application matrix (water), RTLC gave good accuracy which was comparable to LSC. However the variation in the results when small amounts of radioactivity were applied was much larger with RTLC than with LSC.

Preliminary error analysis suggested that this variation was caused mainly by machine error. This suggested that when small amounts of radioactivity (with water as the matrix) were analyzed, strict attention must be paid to keeping all the factors, that may contribute to this variation, as constant as possible. Clearly it will be necessary to investigate these factors to identify the major sources of error.

When larger amounts of radioactivity were applied the variation in the results obtained by RTLC and LSC were comparable and this variation was mainly caused by application errors.

The first of the many factors which might affect the accuracy and reproducibility of the RTLC which we investigated was that of the position of the detector wire. The position (± 3mm) of the detector wire was not critical. The diameter of our spot was approximately 2mm so that when the

Table 5. Comparison of Errors Occurring in Radio-Thin Layer Chromatography

| | Standard Deviations | | | | |
| | | Application | | Total | |
Radioactivity applied (dpm)	Machine (n=80)	Experimental (n=20)	Calculated	No Offset (n=80)	With detector wire offset (exp. 1a) (n=28)
Blank	5.9	3.2	1.5	6.1	5.0
92	14.4	7.6	3.8	14.9	13.6
182	14.7	8.4	5.2	15.6	15.4
633	24.0	31.7	27.9	36.8	26.3
1802	38.8	55.2	47.7	61.5	53.5
7113	89.7	291.0	264.4	279.2	178.9

detector wire was offset by 3mm it was in fact 4mm from the furthest edge of the spot. This implied that any radioactive application anywhere, but completely, within ± 4mm of the detector wire would be analyzed similarly. As the spot or streak size increased up to 8mm the position of the detector wire should become more critical. Obviously further investigation will be required to confirm and delineate this hypothesis.

The second factor we investigated was the matrix, in this case three biological fluids (bile, plasma and urine). The reduction in counts obtained varied not only with different biological fluids but with different dilutions of the same biological fluid. The exact explanation for this reduction was not obtained. However absorption of the radioactivity by the constituents of the biological fluid did not appear to be a major factor. The criterion for the Rf of the constituents was their UV absorption at 220nm. The position of non-UV absorbing constituents was not known and these may or may not affect the results.

The major factor that caused the variation in results appeared to have been variation in the spatial distribution of the radioactive compound. This variation may have occurred during application of the sample or during elution of the plate or both. Furthermore the magnitude of the variation in spatial distribution may be determined by a myriad of factors such as the compound, application solvent, TLC layer, elution solvent, Rf and matrix. Further work would be necessary to identify the exact sources of this variation.

In the introduction we stated that we quoted all our results with the rider that they were only semi-quantitative. From the results of these experiments we have not been persuaded to change this statement.

Although RTLC was quantitative when the sample was applied in a relatively simple matrix, biological matrices did affect the results. Therefore the comparison of results from biological samples, especially comparisons of results from different biological fluids, must be interpreted with caution.

RTLC is a widely used technique which is, superficially, very simple and uncomplicated. With the advent of the new analyzers and their sophisticated software packages there arises the problem that the numbers generated may be interpreted without thought to the limitations of the technique. The results described here show that a certain amount of circumspection should be used when interpreting such data.

REFERENCES

1. S. D. Shulman, J.Liq.Chromatogr., 6:35 (1983).
2. R. Stevenson, Amer.Lab., 49 May (1970).
3. H. Filthuth, Ind.Res.Dev., 23:140 (1981).
4. H. Filthuth, Git.Fachz.Lab., 28:870 (1984).
5. S. Ebel, E. Glaser and D. Rost, High Resolut.Chromatogr.Chromatogr
    Commun., 1:250 (1978).
6. S. J. Constanzo and M. J. Cardone, J.Liq.Chromatogr., 7:2711 (1984).

SOLID PHASE EXTRACTION OF PLASMA FOR METABOLITE
PROFILING BY RADIO-THIN-LAYER CHROMATOGRAPHY

F. A. Tucker

Servier Research and Development
Fulmer Hall, Fulmer
Nr Slough SL3 6HH, UK

SUMMARY

The use of Bond Elut cartridges for solid phase extraction of plasma, prior to drug metabolite profiling by TLC is illustrated here, using a β-blocker (tertatolol) and a xanthine derivative as examples. A simple reversed-phase (C_{18}) extraction was used for the former and for the latter, a cation exchange column (CBA) coupled with protein precipitation. The resulting extracts were free of endogenous materials (e.g. proteins and lipids) and consequently linear analyzer scans of TLC plates showed good resolution between drug and metabolites combined with increased radioactivity on the TLC plate due to the concentration of the sample during extraction. This allowed ease of comparison of metabolites with UV absorbing non-radiolabelled standards and accurate quantitation of metabolite profiles.

INTRODUCTION

Drug metabolism studies routinely involve profiling of ^{14}C labelled drug and its metabolites from plasma. The information gained from this profiling aids identification of pharmacologically active metabolites which may explain a drugs' pharmacology and toxicology in the animal species tested. This profiling can be carried out by thin-layer chromatography (TLC) and subsequent radioscanning on a linear analyzer to locate and quantify metabolites.

Plasma often contains low concentrations of radiolabelled drug-related materials so extraction of up to 5 mls of of sample is needed to facilitate detection of metabolites of interest which may be present at low levels. Also, to obtain good separation of plasma metabolites by TLC, the sample extract applied to the plate needs to be free of endogenous materials such as proteins and lipids.

To achieve this, various plasma extraction methods can be employed. Protein precipitation with alcohol, trichloroacetic acid or acetonitrile is one approach but evaporation of the resulting supernatent can be difficult due to its aqueous content. Liquid-liquid extraction methods are an alternative, but the need for large volumes of extraction solvent often produces a cumbersome method. However, the use of solid phase extraction cartridges enables easy clean up of plasma samples combined with concentration of radiolabelled metabolites into a volatile solvent suitable for application onto a TLC plate.

The results presented below show the application of solid phase extraction as a clean up procedure for plasma metabolite profiling of two drugs, a sulphur containing β-blocker (tertatolol) and a xanthine type derivative, at various times after administration of ^{14}C labelled drug to human volunteers.

METHODS

Plasma samples were obtained from human disposition and metabolism studies using ^{14}C labelled tertatolol (DL-8-(2-hydroxy, 3-t-butylamino-propyloxy)-thiochroman, hydrochloride salt, 5mg/30µCi per subject) and xanthine derivative (120mg/30µCi per subject).

Sample Preparation
Dependent on the level of radioactivity in the plasma, up to 5mls of sample were prepared for extraction as follows:-

Tertatolol: The plasma was diluted with an equal volume of deionized water and spiked with non-radiolabelled UV absorbing standards. These were added at levels of approximately 10µg as a methanol solution (100µl). Centrifugation at 2,500 rpm for 10 minutes sedimented any protein fibres so the supernatent was ready for application to Bond Elut solid phase extraction cartridges (Analytichem Int. Harbor, CA 90710).

Xanthine derivative: Dilution of plasma with an equal volume of 0.1M citrate buffer (PH2.7) precipitated plasma proteins, then centrifugation at 3000 rpm for 15 minutes gave a supernatent suitable for loading directly onto Bond Elut cartridges.

Solvation of Extraction Cartridges

The Bond Elut cartridges were fitted into a vacuum manifold (Vac Elut, Analytichem Int. Harbor, CA 90710).

For extraction of plasma from subjects treated with tertatolol, 3ml C_{18} cartridges were solvated with methanol (3mls) and de-ionized water (3 mls). For extraction of plasma from subjects treated with the xanthine derivative, 1ml CBA (weak cation exchange) and 1ml C_8 cartridges were used 'in tandem' with the CBA first. Solvation of CBA cartridges was with methanol (1ml) followed by 0.1M pH6 citrate buffer (1ml), and for C_8, methanol (1ml) was followed by water (1ml).

Sample Extraction

The sample supernatant was loaded, and a vacuum applied (15-20 in.Hg) to pull the sample through.

For tertatolol, the columns were washed with water (3 x 500µl) and eluted with methanol (2 x 500µl).

For the xanthine derivative, a water wash (2 x 500µl) was followed by methanol elution (2 x 500µl) and 20% ammonia (S.G. 0.88) in methanol (2 x 500µl).

The organic eluates (2mls) were evaporated to dryness under nitrogen and the tertatolol extraction residue dissolved in methanol (50µl) ready

for application to a TLC plate. The xanthine extraction residue was dissolved in methanol (50µl) containing a mixture of non-radiolabelled UV
absorbing standards prior to TLC.

Thin-Layer Chromatography

Each sample was applied as a discrete 15mm band to a Merck Silica gel
60 TLC plate (BDH, Poole, Dorset), using a Linomat IV TLC sample applicator
(Camag, Muttenz, Switzerland).

Solvent systems were:-

Tertatolol

n-Butanol 60: glacial acetic acid 20 : water 20 (v/v).

Xanthine Derivative

Double development:
(i) 1,1,1, Trichloroethane 50 : ethyl acetate 20 : glacial acetic acid 15
     : ethanol 15 (v/v).
(ii) Propan-2-ol 70 : 1,1,1, trichloroethane 20 : water 5 : ammonia 5
     (v/v).

After development the TLC plates were dried and scanned for up to 3 hours
using a Berthold LB284 Linear Analyzer (Laboratory Impex, Twickenham,
Middlesex) prior to autoradiography for 2 months.

RESULTS

Tertatolol Profiles

Plasma volumes extracted using the Bond Elut cartridges were 3, 4 and
5 mls to give 9020 dpm (1 hr), 8702 dpm (4 hr), and 10878 dpm (10 hr)
respectively. The drug metabolite profiles achieved by radioscanning for 3
hours on a linear analyzer are shown in Figure 1. These profiles show the
decrease of the parent drug (D) and increase in a major metabolite (M) over
a 10 hour period. The broadness of the xanthine band suggests the presence
of minor metabolites (X and Y) not resolved by the linear analyzer,
although the chromatography was satisfactory. Subsequent autoradiography
confirmed this.

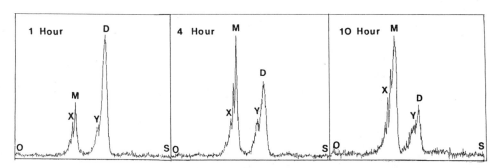

Fig. 1.   Tertatolol drug metabolite profiles at 1, 4 and 10 hours post
dose. D = Drug, M = Major metabolite, X and Y = Minor metabolites,
0 = Origin, S = Solvent front.

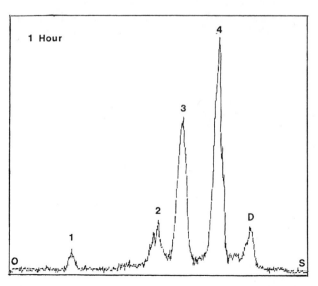

Fig. 2. Xanthine drug metabolite profile at 1 hour post dose. D = Drug,
1 to 4 = Metabolites, O = Origin, S = Solvent.

Xanthine Derivative Profiles

Extraction and TLC of 1 hour (2948 dpm in 2ml) and 4 hour (1200 dpm in 2ml) plasmas followed by radioscanning gave a metabolite profile represented by that in Figure 2.

This profile demonstrates that absorbed parent drug (D) was extensively metabolised even after only 1 hour and this result agrees with HPLC analysis of the parent drug in the samples. The 4 hour plasma profile did not indicate a significant change in metabolite ratios (peaks 1 to 4) from those at 1 hour post dose.

DISCUSSION

The linear analyzer scans of the plasma extracts from each drug (Figures 1 and 2) show clear metabolite profiles, which are consistent across the time periods (Figure 1). Bond Elut extraction minimized the amount of protein and lipid present in the organic extract facilitating its application onto the TLC plate as a neat band allowing successful chromatography without distortion of bands by endogenous materials.

For profiling of tertatolol, plasma was loaded onto a reversed-phase (C_{18}) Bond Elut without prior protein precipitation. The retention of drug related materials was found to be 78.3% (n = 5, CV = 7.9%). This incomplete retention could be due to protein binding of drug related materials inhibiting their affinity for the active sites on the Bond Elut cartridge. Alternatively, competition between drug related materials and endogenous plasma constituents for binding sites may occur, resulting in less than 100% retention. However, the latter is unlikely as recovery was found to be unrelated to plasma volume extracted.

To ensure 100% retention of drug and metabolites from plasma onto the Bond Elut cartridges during xanthine derivative plasma profiling, protein precipitation was introduced into the method.

It has been shown that addition of 30% v/v acetonitrile to plasma destroys the protein conformation but avoids complete protein precipitation and this releases parent drug allowing it to bind fully to a reversed-phase Bond Elut (R. Richards, personal communication). This approach was tried for xanthine derivative plasma profiling, but even at this low level of organic solvent the more polar drug metabolites were being immediately eluted from extraction cartridges on loading.

To overcome this problem, acid protein precipitation in conjunction with a weak cation exchange column and a C_8 reversed-phase column was chosen for xanthine derivative plasma profiling. Theoretically, the use of a pH6 buffer for CBA solvation ensured complete ionization of its carboxylic acid groups such that they were available for cation exchange. Protein precipitation of the sample with pH2.7 0.1M citrate buffer reduced the matrix pH to approximately 5 which allowed ionization of pertinent groups in drug related materials making them available for binding to carboxylic acid moieties on the Bond Elut. The C_8 Bond Elut 'scavenged' any metabolites not held by cation exchange mechanisms. Retention of drug related materials on this system was initially assessed using control blank plasma spiked with ^{14}C radiolabelled parent drug or urine containing radiolabelled metabolites from the same study source as the plasma to be profiled. Retention was found to be 98%.

For both drugs non-radiolabelled ultra violet absorbing standards were included either prior to extraction (tertatolol) or during sample band application (xanthine derivative). The latter is preferable because addition of standards to plasma prior to extraction may mean premature saturation of sites on the extraction cartridges and so reduce retention of drug related material. However, inclusion of standards ensured that chromatographic effects on metabolites by endogenous materials in the plasma were taken into account in chromatography of standards. Bond Elut extraction minimized proteins and lipids from the final extract resulting in profiles clear of UV absorbing materials, so the exact position of putative metabolite standards could be accurately visualized under UV light. The position of these was matched with radioactive bands on linear analyzer scans and autoradiographs to aid in metabolite identification.

For quantification of drug metabolite profiles extraction of up to 5mls of plasma ensured application of sufficient radioactivity to the TLC plate so that the contribution of background radioactivity on the linear analyzer scan was minimal. This enabled accurate quantification of metabolite profiles for each time period.

In conclusion, solid phase extraction allows easy, efficient extraction of up to 5mls of plasma and at the same time removes proteins and lipids so that good clear separation of metabolites occurs during chromatography. Thus, drug metabolite profiles can be easily quantified and the exact position of radioactive bands compared with UV absorbing non-radioactive standards for metabolite identification.

THE USE OF RADIO-THIN LAYER CHROMATOGRAPHY IN

PESTICIDE ENVIRONMENTAL STUDIES

C. R. Leake

Schering Agrochemicals Ltd.
Environmental Science Department
Chesterford Park Research Station
Nr Saffron Walden, Essex UK, CB10 1XL

SUMMARY

All novel pesticides are investigated for their degradation rate and route in the environment prior to obtaining company and government approval to enable sales to proceed.

The incorporation of a radiolabel e.g. ^{14}C, ^{3}H, ^{32}P and ^{125}I into a pesticide molecule enables the selective detection of the molecule and its co-extracted radiolabelled metabolites in the presence of the many compounds that are removed during solvent extraction of samples such as soils, plants and animal tissues.

Radio-thin layer chromatography is a simple but powerful technique for the separation of the radiolabelled compounds present in these extracts for both analytical and preparative work.

Once separated the radiolabelled products can be detected by a variety of techniques only some of them quantitative.

A linear analyzer may be used to obtain a rapid, and relatively sensitive, quantification of the radioactive components on a single track. However, in order to account for losses of volatile components during application and development, plate scraping and scintillation counting is required. The use of a beta-camera provides a two-dimensional picture of the location of the radioactivity on a TLC plate and can be useful in preparative work. Autoradiography, although more time consuming, provides invaluable confirmation of both linear analyzer and beta camera results and acts as a vital aid to co-chromatography problem solving.

Some potential problems of TLC analysis are discussed and a scheme is proposed to overcome them.

INTRODUCTION

Detailed studies are conducted on the decline of the three major classes of compounds namely herbicides, fungicides and insecticides in soils, plants and animals.

107

In order to increase the sensitivity of the limit of detection radio-chemical atoms e.g. carbon 14, tritium and phosphorus 32 may be incorporated into the pesticide molecule.

The use of dual labels may assist the elucidation of the breakdown of separate components of the molecule e.g. Parathion[1] See Figure 1. The radiolabelled pesticide is applied to the soil or plant and then at various times, perhaps up to one year later, the soil or plant is extracted with solvents of increasing polarity, probably terminating with either methanol or acetonitrile/water mixtures. The extracts not only contain the parent pesticide and metabolites but also a large number of co-extracted compounds. From soils these compounds consist of a wide range of organic materials derived from, for example, root exudates, plant decomposition products and microorganisms. One of the major tasks of the pesticide metabolism chemist is to devise appropriate methods to separate the radioactive components of interest from the co-extracted material. One of the most powerful, yet underrated, techniques available to achieve this is radio-thin layer chromatography. In general radio-thin layer chromatography (RTLC) is used with two objectives, firstly the use of analytical TLC to characterize and quantify the proportions of radiolabelled compounds present and secondly preparative (prep) TLC to separate radiolabelled compounds as an initial 'clean-up' prior to further chromatographic investigation e.g. radio-high performance liquid chromatography (HPLC) or gas chromatography mass spectrometry (GC-MS).

It should be borne in mind, however, that for accurate and reproducible TLC the preparation of the solvent tank and elution solvent is critical. TLC tanks should be prepared well in advance and have air-tight seals to retain a saturated atmosphere within[2].

ANALYTICAL TLC

Pesticide transformation pathways are elucidated by the separation and characterization of the products formed. Separation can be achieved using analytical TLC plates which generally have layers about 250 μm thick. Potential metabolites may be chromatographed as standards alongside the extracts, as well as admixed with them in order that their presence in the

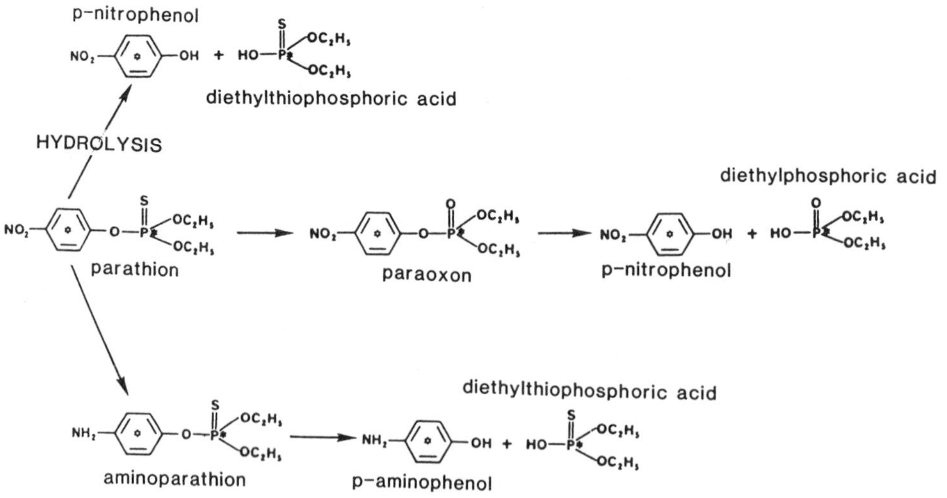

Fig. 1.   Degradation of parathion(1). U-^{14}C radiolabelled, ^{32}P radiolabelled. ☆ ★ indicate position of radiolabels.

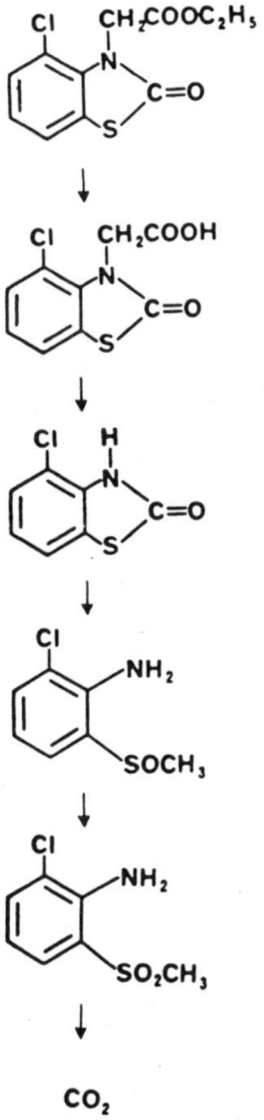

Fig. 2. The degradation of benazolin-ethyl in soil.

extract might be identified. The proportions of each compound present may then be determined using a variety of radiochemical techniques.

The degradation of the herbicide benazolin-ethyl in soil by micro-organisms may be used to illustrate the use of analytical plates. (Figure 2). The metabolites were initially extracted from soil with the non-polar solvent dichloromethane. All five compounds can be separated using Macherey-Nagel, silica gel, TLC plates with a relatively non-polar eluting solvent in this case 2% ethanol stabilized chloroform containing a small proportion (5%) of glacial acetic acid (Figure 3). The addition of acid improves the chromatography of benazolin-acid (pKa 3.65) by suppressing ionization which can cause streaking on the TLC plate. Other organic acids such as formic may also be used. Separations of this type are fairly readily achieved if the original extracting solvent is non-polar e.g. dichloromethane. However, a second extraction of the soil sample with a more polar mixture, such as acetonitrile-water, will remove previously un-extracted radioactive compounds together with more polar co-extracted compounds. These more polar co-extracted compounds can cause retention of radiochemically labelled metabolites on the origin of the TLC plate. See figures 4 and 5.

Such origin material frequently consists of small quantities of radio-active products with higher Rf's which have been 'held back'. This can be overcome in several ways:

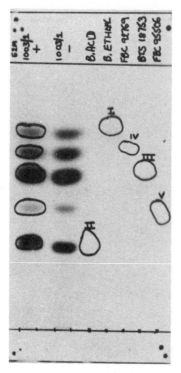

Macherey-Nagel 0.25mm Silica with fluorescent UV254
SOLVENT SYSTEM CHLOROFORM / G.ACETIC ACID   95/5

Fig. 3.   Separation of benazolin-ethyl and soil formed metabolites.

1.   Scraping off the silica at the TLC plate origin, followed by extrac-
     tion into a solvent, concentration and subsequent re-elution under the
     same conditions often shows that non-polar compounds were retained by
     the co-extracted material.

2.   Solid phase extraction onto cartridges such as the Sep-Pack can be
     used to retain the polar material and elute the compounds of interest
     in increasingly polar solvents. When dealing with small quantities of
     unknown compounds it can often be difficult to obtain complete elution
     from the cartridge. It is also difficult to quantify this retained
     material, whereas application of a crude extract to a TLC plate will
     clearly indicate the presence of radiolabelled material remaining on
     the origin.

3.   Different types of silica surface such as concentration zone plates,
     or other media such as cellulose plates or C_{18} chemically bonded
     reversed-phase plates can be utilized. C_{18} chemically bonded
     'reversed-phase' plates with polar solvents have proved successful for
     the chromatography of polar extracts. Results have shown a good
     quantitative agreement between compounds separated by Macherey-Nagel
     normal phase silica and Whatman reversed-phase plates. (Figure 6 and
     Table 1).

     Other types of plates which have been found to be useful include high
performance (HP) TLC plates. Besides increased speed of development
certain compounds which were poorly resolved on analytical plates have been
resolved by HPTLC[3].

110

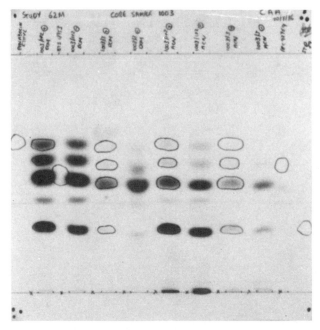

Macherey-Nagel 0.25mm Silica gel with fluorescent indicator UV254

Solvent System : chloroform / G.acetic acid   95/5

Fig. 4.   Comparison of dichloromethane (left) and acetonitrile (right)
extracts of soil cores.

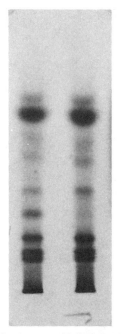

Flooded soil extracted with dichloromethane

Fig. 5.   Rechromatography of radiolabelled metabolites recovered from the
origin of a silica gel TLC plate (see Figure 4).

Normal phase   Reverse phase

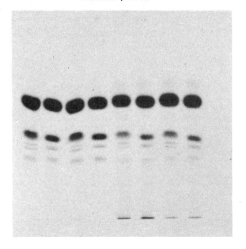
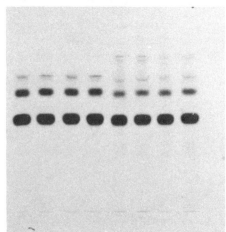

Macherey Nagel 0.25 mm silica gel   Whatman KC18F 0.2 mm C18bonded silica
with fluorescent indicator UV254   with fluorescent indicator UV254

Solvent system :   Solvent system :
Chloroform/Ethanol/G.Acetic acid   Acetonitrile/Water 80/20
95/5/1

Fig. 6.   Comparison of chromatography of polar metabolites on normal and
           reversed-phase TLC plates.

Table 1.   Polar Solvent Extract. Acetonitrile/water 80/20.

Plate type	Macherey-Nagel Silica F254		Whatman KC 18F	
Solvent System	Chloroform/Absolute Alcohol/ Glacial Acetic acid 95/5/1 v/v		Acetonitrile/water 4/1 v/v	
Component	% Component Detected			
	+	–	+	–
Compound A	88.6	89.3	87.1	88.5
Compound B	6.5	6.1	7.2	6.9
Remainder	3.1	3.0	2.9	2.4
Unknowns	1.8	1.5	2.7	2.2
Total	100.0	100.0	100.0	100.0

+ indicates added non-radiolabelled compound.
– indicates neat extracts.

Results obtained by Linear analyzer

     The detection of radiolabelled compounds can be achieved using several
techniques. The Linear analyzer provides a relatively sensitive detection
system within a 2 cm x 20 cm track and it is possible to detect below 100
dpm of ^{14}C in a single band[4]. However, it is sometimes difficult to
observe minor compounds in the presence of one or two major compounds and
if co-chromatography is taking place no clue is provided by the one dimensional printout.

Table 2. Comparison between Linear Analyzer and Plate Scraping

Sample	% A		% B		% Unknowns		% Remainder	
	Linear analyzer	Scraping	Linear analyzer	Scraping	Linear analyzer	Scraping	Linear analyzer	Scraping
2025 +	75.9	75.5	20.6	21.5	1.1	2.9	2.5	0.1
2025 −	77.5	76.1	19.7	20.7	0.8	3.0	2.0	0.1
2039 +	86.2	85.2	10.9	11.8	2.7	3.0	0.2	0.1
2039 −	86.2	85.4	11.0	11.5	2.2	3.0	0.7	0.2
2052 +	87.5	85.4	10.3	10.8	2.2	3.8	0.0	0.0
2052 −	87.6	85.4	10.9	10.4	1.5	4.2	0.1	0.0

+ indicates added non radiolabelled compound
− indicates neat extract

Comparisons between linear analyzer and plate scraping and scintillation counting are generally good even when a proportion of the radioactivity remains on the origin. (Table 2).

However problems are more likely to be encountered with minor components (<5% of total). The difficulty with plate scraping is ensuring the removal of radioactivity from the silica in the scintillation cocktail though the addition of methanol and other solvents can assist this. Total recovery from the plate is only assured using plate scraping – in order to confirm that there are no losses due to volatile compounds. Autoradiography provides a valuable 2-dimensional picture and may be used to differentiate minor compounds which would not be fully resolved in a linear analyzer printout – however it does not provide a quantitative result of the proportions of compounds on the plate. Some workers have reported densitometer evaluations, however X-ray film has a low dynamic range and it is very easy to over expose the film with a major band. A combination of techniques is therefore required – quantification of some plates by plate scraping and scintillation counting in order to validate linear analyzer results, followed by autoradiography in order to assist linear analyzer evaluation and a guide to co-chromatography problem solving. A Spark Chamber provides a quick 2-dimensional picture which can be useful in prep TLC.

PREP-TLC

In general the ability of a prep-TLC plate to separate larger quantities of compounds increases as the square root of the thickness of the layer, thus a 1000 μm layer will have twice the load capacity of a 250 μm (analytical) plate. Thus, using a 2000 μm plate, which is about the maximum recommended thickness, up to 500 mg may be separated according to the separation characteristics. One use is to separate minor metabolites from a mixture in order to obtain sufficient quantity in a reasonably pure state for mass spectrometry. However it is not always possible to directly transfer the separation from analytical plates to prep-scale – see Figure 7. The location of the bands may be observed by using a Spark Chamber. The image obtained can be projected back onto the plate in order to clearly define the separate areas or autoradiography may be used. The appropriate band (including the polar origin material if desired) may then be removed and the compound extracted from the silica into a suitable solvent. Methanol is not recommended as it dissolves silica which may then precipitate on concentration. Most of the commonly used solvents e.g. acetone, ethyl-acetate, dichloromethane, or the more polar ethanol will not dissolve the fluorescent additive which enables the use of non-radiolabelled standards as marker compounds run along side the sample.

If problems are encountered then plates without the fluorescent in-dicator should be used and the standards visualized by spray reagents (preferably non-reactive ones e.g. Iodine vapor). Washing the plates by pre-eluting with methanol can help to remove some impurities in the silica. It is also possible to 'pre-activate' the plates by drying or eluting with another solvent.

If a large number of TLC plates are required in order to generate sufficient quantity of material it may be cost effective to develop a prep-HPLC system, however problems may be encountered if there is a large amount of polar material present or if the compounds are difficult to partition from water based mobile phase which would be unsuitable for gas chromatography - mass spectrometry.

Potential pitfalls in the use of TLC

Although TLC is an apparently straight forward technique a number of potential problems and artefacts have been observed in our laboratories

1. Thermal degradation:-
   The use of warm air hair driers to speed up solvent evaporation during application to the plate surface has caused thermal degradation on the TLC plate.

2. Volatilization from TLC plates:-
   Compounds with a high vapor pressure are readily lost from TLC plates. For example 2,4,6-trichlorophenol is subject to this type of behavior.

ANALYTICAL   PREP.

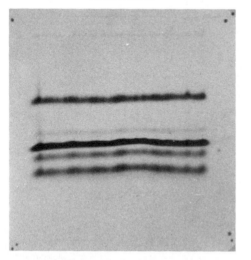 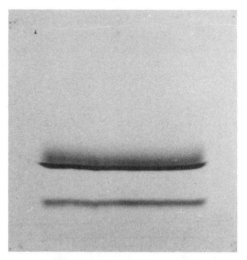

Macherey Nagel 0.25 mm silica gel   Macherey Nagel 2.00mm silica gel
with fluorescent indicator UV254   with fluorescent indicator UV254

solvent system: chloroform / g.acetic acid 95/5

Fig. 7. Comparison of separation on analytical and preparative plates.

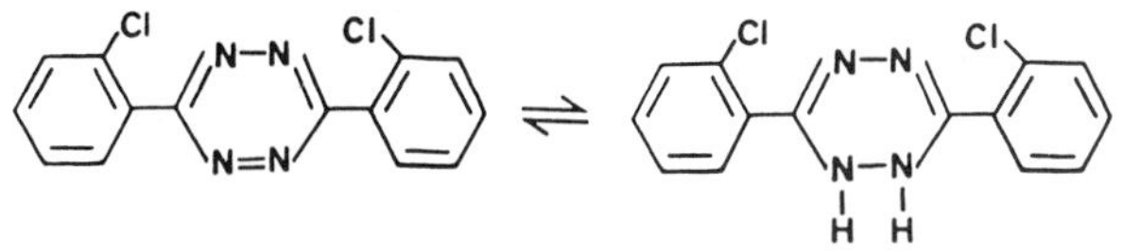

Fig. 8. Oxidised (left) and reduced (right) forms of the acaricide
NC21314.

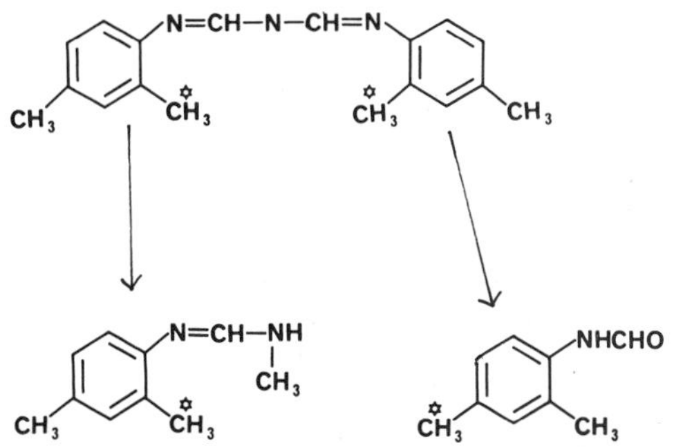

Fig. 9. Degradation of amitraz on silica gel TLC plates.

3. Reduction/oxidation reactions:-
Reduction or oxidation reactions may take place on the silica surface.
This can be caused by the addition of potential metabolites which may
cause reduction of compounds in the plant or soil extract. For
example the addition of the potential metabolite NC 22505 to extracts
containing the radiolabelled acaricide NC 21314 resulted in the
formation of radiolabelled NC 22505 on the plate (Figure 8).

4. Instability on silica surface:-
Some compounds can decompose on the silica surface and it was found
that the breakdown of the compound amitraz during a purity determination was prevented by using concentration zone plates. On normal
silica surface degradation of the compound occurred. The proposed
scheme for the decomposition of this compound on silica gel is shown
in Figure 9.

Proposed scheme for the characterization by radio-thin layer chromatography
of pesticide metabolites

     The radio-labelled extracts should be divided into two equal portions,
one portion admixed with non-radiolabelled potential metabolites. Each
portion is applied to the TLC plate separately as a narrow 1 cm band using
a mechanical applicator if possible. It is important to ensure that a
layer of sample is not accumulated above the silica layer as this will
cause streaking. The potential metabolites should be spotted separately on
the plate so that any oxidation or interconversion can be observed. The
plate is then developed in a sealed tank. The recovery of radioactivity
from the plate needs to be checked by plate scraping and scintillation
counting. If the potential metabolite is genuine then an isotopic dilution
effect will be observed and the radioactive component will be seen to fill
the whole of the ultraviolet quenched area. If the radioactivity does not
fill the whole area then it is possible that co-chromatography is taking
place. Additionally 2-D TLC can be used to confirm identity. Normally

each extract ought to be examined using a minimum of two types of TLC plate in separate solvent systems, with several being used in the method development stage.

Thin-layer chromatography is a powerful technique in metabolism chemistry and when used properly can produce valid and accurate results.

ACKNOWLEDGEMENT

I would like to thank my colleagues at Schering Agrochemicals in particular Mr. D. Arnold, Mr. I. Morton and Miss. S. Newby for their help in the preparation of this paper.

REFERENCES

1.   S. U. Kahn, in: "Pesticides in the Soil Environment," Elsevier, Amsterdam, p.114 (1980).
2.   E. Stahl, "Thin Layer Chromatography - A Laboratory Handbook," Springer Verlag, Berlin (1965).
3.   J. C. Touchstone, "Advances in Thin Layer Chromatography Clinical and Environmental Applications," John Wiley and Son, Chichester (1982).
4.   H. Filthuth, in: "Analytical and Chromatographic Techniques in Radio-pharmaceutical Chemistry," D. M. Wieland, M. C. Tobes, and T. J. Mangner, (eds.), Springer Verlag, New York, p. 79 (1986).

A NOTE ON: DEVELOPMENT OF 2-DIMENSIONAL DETECTORS FOR

RADIO-THIN-LAYER CHROMATOGRAPHY

G. Dietzel, H. Kubisiak and H. Stelzer

Raytest
Benz Strasse 3, 7541, Straubenhardt 1
W. Germany

SUMMARY

The development of a series of detectors for planar radio-chromatography is described (sensitivities are quoted as dpm of carbon-14). The RITA is a position sensitive proportional counter with a resolution of 0.5mm and a sensitivity of a few tens of dpm. This detector may be used, with suitable software, to analyze two dimensional thin-layer chromatography (TLC) plates. TRACY is a multiwire proportional detector which has been developed especially for two dimensional planar chromatography. This detector has a resolution of 1mm with a sensitivity of about 25dpm for an analysis time of 15 minutes. BERTA is a spark chamber which also has been developed for two dimenional radio-detection. The spark chamber has a resolution of 1mm with a sensitivity of about 10dpm in 40 minutes. One of the major disadvantages of such spark chambers has been the lack of any digital information. This has been solved by development of EVA, an optical reading system for the BERTA where a special diode array matrix is used in conjunction with a very fast Motorola 68000 CPU.

INTRODUCTION

In discussing the design of instruments for the determination of the distribution of radioactivity in 2-dimensions on a TLC plate a brief history of the development of the field may be useful.

Thus in 1962 Schulze and Wenzel[1] described a windowless proportional gas flow-through detector for the measurement of tritium (^{3}H) and carbon-14 (^{14}C) on TLC plates (the patent application having been made in December, 1961).

Then in 1965, in Vienna, F. Berthold[2] reported the use of the Schulze and Wenzel detector for 2-dimensional TLC. The open window of the detector was only a few millimetres wide and the detector had to be moved over the entire TLC track in a meander pattern. A dot printer, mounted in parallel with the detector, plotted a small line for a selectable number of counts detected. A high number of dots per area symbolized a high local activity. In this way a coarse picture, comparable to an autoradiogram, was created. The resolution was about 5mm and the sensitivity for ^{3}H was good and was indeed comparable with autoradiography. In this way a two

117

dimensional picture of a TLC plate could be obtained within a day or overnight. This was much faster than the 3 to 6 weeks waiting for the exposure
of an autoradiogram. However at that time a digital evaluation of the 2-
dimensional picture was not possible.

The development of various types of gas counting tubes can be divided
into two separate schools epitomised by Charpak and Borkowski.

In 1968 Charpak[3] reviewed the evaluation of spark chambers and
discussed the various types available and their development. He also
discussed the development of multiwire proportional counters (MPC). He was
of the opinion that the analysis of low energy radiation could be achieved
much more simply using multiwire proportional counters than with spark
chambers.

Charpak also stated that the lower limit of the particle energy at
which the technique would be useful was a function of the window thickness
of the detector. As soon as a particle lost an ion-pair in the gas envel-
ope the particle could be detected. The idea was taken up by Numelec
(Paris) who wanted Charpak to provide a design for a TLC radio chromat-
agrahic detector (personal communication).

At the beginning of 1977 Numelec introduced their "Type Charpak"
Chromelec radio-chromatographic detector. This was the first commercially
available instrument and was able to read a 10 x 200mm TLC track using a
one dimensional position sensitive proportional counter.

In March 1974 Gabriel and Bram[4] had reported 1-dimensional measurements of ^{14}C electrophoerograms. The chamber was 10mm high, 25mm wide and
250mm long with a 25 micrometer thick window. They suggested that their
linear counter might be adapted to measure low energy electrons from ^{3}H by
using a very thin entrance window. In April 1974 Bram[5] filed for a
patent for "a method and apparatus designed for the purpose of quickly
determining with high resolution, the spatial distribution of radioactivity
of an object emitting radioactive particles, especially those of low
energy".

For ^{3}H the TLC plate or other object was enclosed within a chamber
which could be pressurized by a counting gas. For ^{14}C the TLC plate or
other object was placed outside the detector and a 25 micrometer thick
window was used. A two or three dimensional picture of the spatial distribution of radioactivity could be obtained with this detector. We believe
that the Bram patent(s) can be related back to Charpaks[3] original idea in
1968.

Gabriel and Bram[4] refer to Brokowski and Kopp[6] who had already
developed and obtained a patent for a one dimensional position sensitive
proportional counter in May 1968. In 1970 Borkowski and Kopp[7] reported
on some applications and properties of one and two dimensional counters.
Then in 1972 Borkowski and Kopp used their instrument to analyze ^{14}C
material on a TLC plate (personal communication) for a biologist colleague.
After a short period of time a two dimensional picture of nine distinct
radioactive components was obtained on the screen of a storage oscilloscope
(a hard copy of the image was made). However, as Borkowski and Kopp only
did basic research on detector developments and were not interested in
curious applications such as radio-TLC the idea was forgotten.

Development of a One Dimensional Detector - RITA

When developing our first position sensitive proportional counter we
took a design similar to the one described by Flynn et al.,[7] and replaced

the large delay line by a flat one after Fisher et al.,[8]. We also
learned from Flynn that particles which enter the detector at an angle of
45° result in reduced resolution compared to those entering perpendicularly. As particles with an angle of 45° have a longer path length in
a flat detector, compared with the perpendicular particles, they generate a
higher pulse. However, by using the energy gates of Flynn those particles
which enter the detector at an angle other than perpendicularly could be
eliminated.

The RITA detector can be used with a collimator, thin window or completely open. The resolution is about 0.5mm for ^{3}H and ^{14}C with a sensitivity of a few tens of dpm for an analysis time of 10 minutes. The homogeneity of the detector is ± 5% and is linear over a range of 5 decades of
radioactivity. The detector head can be moved in steps of 1mm upwards.
The real time multi-task program allows a series of measurements to be made
in the "background" whilst the user operates the system for the pre-
selection of other runs, or evaluations, in the "foreground".

Use of the One Dimensional Detector For Two Dimensional TLC

For two dimensional TLC measurements the RITA can take one dimensional
measurements every 2.5mm and store 77 runs on one disc. The three dimensional display program allows individual selection of every single trace or
all traces at once to build up a three dimensional picture in less than 3
minutes. The three dimensional picture can be tilted between 0 and 90
degrees and turned by up to 180 degrees. This picture can then be printed
on a standard matrix printer within 2 minutes. At any position regions of
interest can be selected in the first trace and projected in the Z-
direction. The integral values of every trace can be plotted against Z.
In this way a one dimensional chromatogram is created in the Z-direction.
The integral values of very trace can be plotted against Z. In this way a
one dimensional chromatogram is created in the Z-direction. If one takes a
sufficient number of steps the resolution can be as fine as the diaphram of
the detector is wide. In principle the width of the diaphram could be as
little as 1mm. However, the user has to make a compromise between the
required resolution and the desired sensitivity. Thus measurement for a
period of one minute at very trace position, would take 77 minutes. The
detection limit would be a few hundred dpm per spot. The advantage of the
RITA is that a machine which was mainly developed for the most efficient
measurement of one dimensional TLC traces can also generate a two dimensional picture. The disadvantage is that the resolution in the Z-direction
is never as good as in the X-direction and therefore the resolution of a
two dimensional picture is not symmetrical.

Development of a Two Dimensional Multiwire Proportional Detector - TRACY

In 1980 Petersen et al.,[10] described a multistep chamber for use as
a detector for radiochromatography imaging. The bidimensional display of
this multiwire proportional counter was performed by the center of gravity
method. We used the idea of the preamplifying gap in front of the counter
and, as we had more experience with such position determination electronics
as a result of our work with the RITA, combined it with the bidimensional
display method of Perez-Mendez[11]. In co-operation with Dr. A. Stelzer a
two dimensional radiochromatographic detector (TRACY) for ^{3}H and ^{14}C was
developed. The detector was incorporated within a vacuum chamber. Inserting a TLC plate, evacuating and refilling with a small amount of counting
gas (argon/methane; 90/10) is a simple operation requiring 2 to 3 minutes.
When completed the system is ready for use. The co-ordinates of the beta
particles that are detected are transferred to an IBM-AT computer and
displayed on the screen. The operator can observe the growing density of
the collected events. After a preset time or count a number of evaluation

programs can be used (e.g. background subtraction). A typical analysis time would be approximately 15 minutes with spots having 25 - 1200 dpm of ^{14}C with a resolution of about 1mm. Two cursors can enclose a region of interest and make a projection on the X- or '-axis. The plot program will generate a 1:1 plot for the entire 200 x 200mm area. An actual measurement is shown in Figure 1 and the autoradiograph of the same TLC plate is shown in Figure 2.

Development of a Two Dimensional Spark Chamber - BERTA

In 1966 Pullan[12] reported the development of a crossed wire spark chamber which was able to analyze ^{14}C on TLC plates with a resolution of about 5mm. However, he also reported that crossed wire spark chambers had proven to be unstable when used for radiochromatography.

Then in 1975 Pullan[13] reported the design, construction and operation of a spark chamber for radiochromatography which used a spiral shaped cathode. However, in our opinion, the spiral shaped cathode does not give good resolution; Pullan reported a resolution 6mm for ^{14}C and 3mm for ^{3}H.

In a review by Roberts[14] in 1978 concerning radiochromatographic instruments three spark chambers were mentioned. None of these instruments had been a commercial success, there are, in our opinion, three major problems which make the spark chamber generally unacceptable and therefore not widely used;

1. difficulties in the homogeneity over the entire chamber.
2. problems of obtaining reproducible results.
3. very high level of maintenance and skill required to keep one detector working (requires a physicist to operate it).

However, one of our customers had gained a lot of experience using several commercially available spark chambers for radio-TLC and found only one type which was reliable enough for his routine laboratory work. The development and manufacture of BERTA was based on his experiences combined

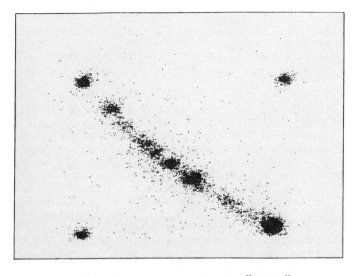

Fig. 1. Measurement taken by "TRACY".

120

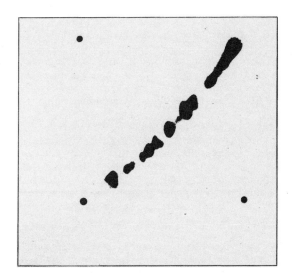

Fig. 2. Autoradiograph of a radio chromatograph (see Figure 1).

with a very detailed literature search in order to determine the problems associated with this approach.

The resulting design (Figure 3) used a fine grid as the anode and cathode planes. These were mounted in parallel and 4mm apart. The grid was made from a woven mesh of stainless steel wires with a diameter of 35mm and a mesh size of 200mm. The mesh structure of the anode and cathode planes has three major advantages:

1. excellent uniformity of the electrical field.
2. a collimation effect.
3. a gas pre-amplification effect in the gaps of the mesh.

The counting gas was a mixture of neon and helium (70:30). A few per cent of ethanol vapor was added to the gas, at a precisely stabilized temperature, to ensure optimal and reproducible working conditions. The design of the BERTA detector results in a detector which is simple to use and very easy to maintain. The detector slides out, like a drawer, for replacement and can be easily disassembled and cleaned. The sample is also placed in a drawer-like mechanism which allows the sample plate to be brought very close and in parallel to the very thin mylar window. The

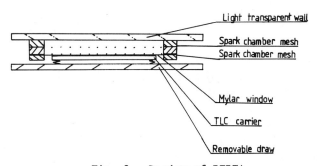

Fig. 3. Design of BERTA.

resolution of the detector is approximately 1mm with a sensitivity of about 10 dpm counted in approximately 40 minutes.

Development of an Optical Reading System for the BERTA – EVA

The main reason for the failure of spark chambers used for radio-TLC was the lack of digital information. A photographic image offers no basis for chromatogram evaluation. EVA, an optical reading system, was developed for use with the BERTA in order to overcome this problem.

A special diode array matrix (576 x 384 sensors) registers every spark event. To evaluate the large amount of data produced a very fast computer with a huge memory capacity is required. The CPU Motorola 68000 (16 bit data, 32 bit instructions) with a VME-bus system was therefore chosen. This allowed extension of the memory capacity of the EVA to 4 Megabytes. In addition, EVA has two 3.5 inch disc drives each with a capacity of 1 Megabyte. The 14 inch color monitor has a resolution of 0.36mm per pixle and can display up to eight colors.

The software enables the presentation of a real time display on the screen as the sparks are collected. The intensity scale (i.e. the number of events per pixle) extends from 0 to 56000 and is represented by the eight different colors. The color ranges are defined by the operator. EVA is controlled by a computer-mouse and all operations and programs available for that particular screen are displayed as a list at the right hand side of the screen. Any number of background counts may be subtracted over the entire screen. Regions of interest may be defined using the mouse and these may be displayed separately or in combinations. All of the regions can be integrated and the results displayed, digitally, at the lower right hand side of the screen. With a normal one dimensional chromatogram rectangular regions of interest may be defined using the mouse. This region will then contain the same information as we would obtain by using the RITA to analyze a single TLC trace. Obviously this allows us to measure many one dimensional traces simultaneously resulting in a great saving of time. Operations such as smoothing, peak search, integration, background subtraction and per cent fraction calculations are standard features. The ability to generate a three dimensional display is another available feature. The three dimensional picture can be tilted and turned to allow the operator the best possible view of the chromatogram.

REFERENCES

1. P. E. Schulze and M. Wenzel, Angew.Chem.Int.Edn., 1:580 (1962).
2. F. Berthold, Proceedings of Symposium on Radioisotope Sample Measurement Techniques in Medicine and Biology, IAEA, Vienna, 303 (1965).
3. G. Charpak, Proceedings of International Symposium on Nuclear Electronics, Versailles (1968).
4. A. Gabriel and S. Bram, FEBS Lett., 39: 307 (1974).
5. S. Bram, French Patent FR 2279114 19.03.76 Priority date: 25.04.74 74 FR-014453.
6. C. J. Borkowski and M. K. Kopp, Rev.Sci.Instrum., 39:1515 (1968).
7. C. J. Borkowski and M. K. Kopp, IEEE Trans.Nucl.Sci., 17:340 (1970).
8. E. R. Flynn, S. Orbesen, N. Stein, H. Thiessen, D. M. Lee, and S. E. Sabottka, Nuclear Instruments and Methods, 111:67 (1973).
9. J. Fisher, H. Okuno, and A. H. Walenta, Nuclear Instruments and Methods, 151:451 (1978).
10. G. Peterson, G. Charpak, G. Melchart, and F. Sauli, Nuclear Instruments and Methods, 176:239 (1980).
11. V. Perez-Mendez, Proceedings of International Meeting on Proportional and Drift Chambers, Dubna USSR, (1975).

12. B. R. Pullan, R. Howard, and B. J. Perry, Nucleonics 72, (1966).
13. B. R. Pullan and J. J. P. De Lima, Nuclear Instruments and Methods, 124:149 (1975).
14. T. R. Roberts, Radiochromatography (J.Chromatogr library, 41), Elsevier/North Holland Biomedical Press, New York and Amsterdam (1978)

A NOTE ON -DIGITAL AUTORADIOGRAPH: A NEW DETECTOR FOR

RADIOCHROMATOGRAPHY AND ELECTROPHORESIS

H. Filthuth

Labor. Prof. Dr. Berthold
7547 Wildbad, FRG

INTRODUCTION

A new detector has been developed, which can measure the 1- and 2-dimensional distribution of ionizing radiation from radioisotopes present on thin-layer chromatography (TLC) plates, electrophoresis gels or indeed any surface distribution of ionizing radiation, (i.e. protein distributions, blots, DNA-sequences, tissue sections).

The detector is a position sensitive multiwire chamber with delay line read-out, detecting with very high sensitivity and high spatial resolution compounds labelled with ^{3}H, ^{125}I, ^{14}C, ^{32}P. Also gamma rays can be detected i.e. from ^{99}Tc and ^{123}I, being converted into electrons by photo – and compton – effects inside the counter.

Beta-particles and gamma-rays emitted from the chromatogram enter the counter from the bottom through an open entrance window of 250mm length and variable width (1m to 25mm). The position (x,y) of an ionizing particle emitted from the object plane (i.e. TLC plates) entering the detector is determined by measuring the projected position y of the counting wire and in measuring the time of propagation T of the pulse signal generated at the counting wire and transmitted into the delay line being proportional to the position x (see Figure 1). After appropriate electronic processing the signals are transmitted to the data acquisition system, an IBM-AT computer or some equivalent.

One-dimensional distributions, Radiochromatograms for TLC plates developed in one direction are detected by placing the chamber directly above the appropriate track.

Following data acquisition, an automatic peak search can be performed. Peak fitting is done by a Gaussian fit method. This allows overlapping peaks to be deconvoluted, resulting in an accurate representation of peak area, the background being automatically subtracted.

Many overlapping peaks which cannot be resolved by the standard "drop line" method can be identified and quantified. The results of the peak fitting and deconvolution can then be printed out in a Gaussian curve format. This represents a dramatically improved method of evaluating and viewing the raw data.

125

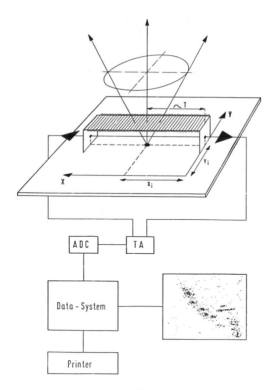

Fig. 1.   Principle of digital autoradiograph.

Bar graphs which translate the area of each peak into a relative height display are also produced. An example of this type of data analysis is shown in Figure 2.

Two-Dimensional Chromatograms

Two dimensional (2D) chromatograms are evaluated by measuring in sequence and small steps down to 1mm using up to several hundred lanes of the TLC plate or gel. The data acquisition system can be used to display and produce a 1:1 scale hard copy from the acquired data, a 2-dimensional representation of the radioactivity present on the plate. This distribution, the <u>digital</u> <u>autoradiograph</u> is quantitative with a large dynamic range (1:320000 per 0.025 mm^2), compared to the very limited dynamic range (1:10) of classical autoradiography using X-Ray film.

Thus the computer analysis of the data goes far beyond the limitations of conventional autoradiography.

The two dimensional analysis procedures can also include contrast enhancement and background subtraction. This allows the selective suppression of the background activity on the plate which leads to higher resolution of the individual spots.

By careful selection of the dynamic range used for evaluation areas of radioactivity can be detected which would normally be overlooked in autoradiography, due to the limited dynamic range of photographic film.

The radioactivity plot of the plate may be presented so that the "optical density" (degree of blackening) is a linear, logarithmic or square-root function of the radioactivity (Figure 3).

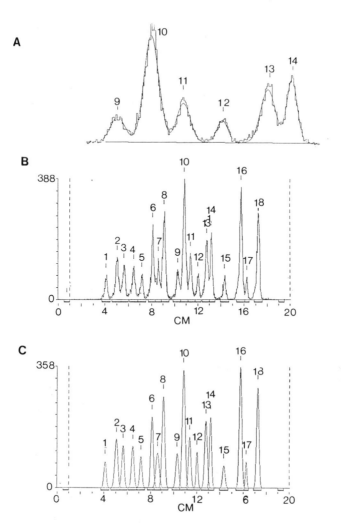

Fig. 2. Data of measured chromatogram with automatic peak search (a) and
         Gaussian fit (b, c).

Analysis of Specific Chromatograms

     By positioning a cursor on selected spots on the two dimensional
display, one may display and work with any individual chromatogram present
on the plate, using all of the one dimensional software features. In this
way one can also linearize any 2-dimensional distribution (Figure 4).

     By setting two cursor pairs around each specific spot the two dimen-
sional program can define an ellipse corresponding to the area within the
cursors. The activity contained within the ellipse may be calculated and
expressed on the integration report as a percent of total activity present
on the plate or as a percent only, the total activity within the integrated
areas (ROI).

     A 3-dimensional radiation distribution of the sample can be generated
from the data, i.e. in the x-y plane the position of the radiating spot in
the z-direction and amount of radiation emitted from this spot. The x-y
plane can be "viewed" at any angle and from any distance (Figure 5).

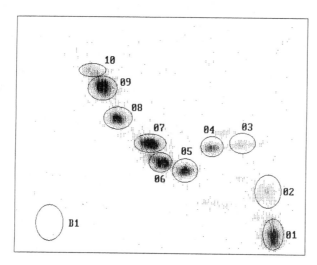

Fig. 3.   Integrated spots with elliptical boundaries on the same
          chromatogram.

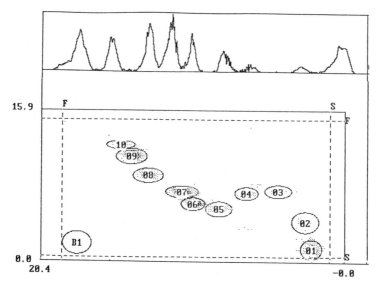

Fig. 4.   Linearization of a 2-dimensional chromatogram.

The detection efficiency of the system is very high. Typically 1,000
dpm of ^{14}C from a TLC-plate (250 micron thick) can be detected in 1 minute
per lane, and a TLC-plate of 20 cm x 20 cm with spot activities of 1000 dpm
^{14}C or more can be measured completely within about 60 minutes. The
spatial resolution of the detecting system is very high. In 2- and 3-
dimensional distributions very close spots or overlapping spots can be
recognized much more easily than in linear distributions. Separations down
to 1 mm can be detected.

CONCLUSIONS

The development of this instrument offers a powerful new tool for the
measurement and analysis of TLC radiochromatography, the detection of

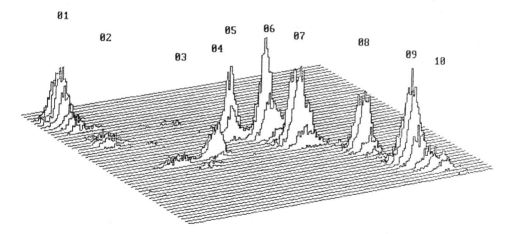

Fig. 5.   3-dimensional display of a 2-d chromatogram.

radioisotope labelled electropherograms and blot distributions. Any surface distribution of ionizing radiation can be detected and measured
quantitatively with high efficiency. Applications of the instrument are
not limited to chromatography, thus for example the distribution of radioactivity in cell cultures and within tissue sections may also be determined. Examples of typical applications have been described elsewhere (see
also Smith, this vol.).

REFERENCES

1.   H. Filthuth, in <u>Proceedings of Second International Symposium, kansas
     City</u>, R.R. Muccino (ed.), Elsevier Science Publishers, B.V.
     Amsterdam, 465 (1986).
2.   H. Filthuth, in <u>Analytical and Chromatographic Techniques in
     Radiopharmaceutical Chemistry</u>, Donald M. Wieland, Michael C.
     Tobes, Thomas J. Mangner, (eds.), Springer Verlag, New York,
     Berlin, Heidelberg, Tokyo, 79 (1986).

A NOTE ON: ADVERSE ELECTROSTATIC EFFECTS SEEN IN RADIO-THIN

LAYER CHROMATOGRAPHY USING A LINEAR ANALYZER

Stephen R. Moss

ICI Plc., Pharmaceuticals Div. Mereside
Alderley Park, Macclesfield
Cheshire, SK10 4TG

INTRODUCTION

Radio thin-layer chromatography (TLC) is used extensively in drug
metabolism studies to provide quantitative information on the metabolic
fate of radiolabelled compounds. Radio-TLC analyzers are the instruments
of choice for this purpose and are basically gas-ionisation detectors with
a positional element (the delay line) that can analyze a whole track at a
time (see, for example. Filthuth 1986[1] for a description of the design of
such instruments).

During the course of routine drug metabolism studies we observed
effects, probably due to a build-up of static electricity, on an Isomess
(Raytest) RITA with an unscreened aperture which adversely affected quantification.

A variety of methods for eliminating this static electricity were
investigated including sprays, plate dampening and earthing strips. However, any improvements were small and temporary.

Here we briefly describe methods of assessing and attenuating this
effect and also of eliminating it (but with concomitant losses in sensitivity and resolution).

EXPERIMENTAL PROCEDURES

The work described below was performed on an Isomess (Raytest) RITA
linear analyzer with Apple IIe data system. The instrument was calibrated
for linearity of response along the detector and for high resolution with
each aperture used.

The TLC plates used were 0.25 mm thick Merck Kieselgel 60 F-254. They
were pre-run in methanol/water (9:1 v/v) and allowed to dry naturally.
Experiments were also carried out to see the effect of drying on susceptability to static build-up by repeatedly scanning a plate and noting the
change in count rate.

The same radioactive source was used throughout these studies. It was
a single spot source of ^{14}C glucose in ink.

RESULTS AND DISCUSSION

The Effect of Drying Time on Static Build-Up

Freshly eluted plates should not be analyzed by instruments with open apertures as damage may be caused to the detector or the delay line due to solvent vapor, especially if acids or alkalis are used in the developing solvent. However, when studies were carried out using neutral aqueous TLC systems the freshly eluted plates initially showed no adverse effects due to static build-up. However, as the plates dried in the gas stream under the detector an increase in susceptability to static was observed. Stable analyzing conditions were only achieved after approximately 6 hours of normal air drying. After this time a plate could be considered to be dry and gave a constant response thereafter.

Thus for a constant response we have demonstrated that "wet" plates should not be analyzed and that "dry" plates are acceptable. Once dry further ageing does not change a plate's susceptability to static build-up.

The Effect of Static Build-Up on Peak Shape

The electrons produced by the gas-ionisation are "mopped-up" by the detector wire (anode) leaving the positive ions to "fall" to the surface of the TLC plate. All our work was performed on silica plates and, as silica is a good insulator, a charge built up which interfered with the field in the detector (the effect is not seen on metal test plates). The resulting effect is represented in Figure 1. Thus, whilst the increase in total counts and peak height should have been directly proportional to the analysis time, with static build-up this was not the case (Table 1). Peaks were shorter and wider and the total counts were lower than those anticipated on the basis of a short analysis time.

The broadening of peaks obtained under conditions where static has built up on a plate has obvious consequences in terms of reducing the resolution of the instrument (as opposed to chromatographic resolution) in that peaks that are close to each other will tend to merge.

There are a number of ways of expressing resolution. These include "peak width at half peak height" which requires measurements to be made from the traces and "peak trough to height ratio" which requires measurements and 2 equal sources (Figure 2). The analyzer acquires data in 1024 channels along the detector and the counts accumulated in the single high-

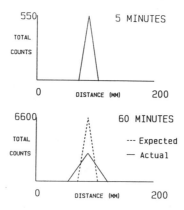

Fig. 1. The effect of static build-up on peak shape with increased analysis time.

Table 1. Isomess Rita (Original) Open Detector Window

Time (secs)	Total counts (C)	Peak max. (M)	$\dfrac{C}{M}$	CPM
60	1979	105	18.8	1979
120	4009	210	19.1	2005
300	10070	550	18.3	2104
600	19497	890	21.9	1950
1200	33737	1350	25.0	1687
2400	58605	2000	29.3	1465
3600	82444	2600	31.7	1374
7200	154496	4600	33.6	1287

est channel (maximum channel count – M) can easily be displayed on the trace. Also readily available from the trace are the total counts in a peak (C). If a single source is used the ratio of C/M gives an assessment of peak shape – the smaller this number then the better the peak shape. This number is only comparable when the exact same source is used. For these studies the C/M ratio was used to assess the quality of the results obtained under a variety of experimental conditions.

The results of one set of measurements made with the standard un-screened aperture are shown in the Table. As the analysis time increased the count rate (counts per minute, cpm) decreased and the C/M ratio increased, demonstrating static build-up.

If the instrument was used for analyzing high activity sources requiring short analysis times or if it was used where good instrumental resolution was not an essential requirement then the problem was less significant. If, however, low activity sources or low energy sources (e.g. ^{3}H) are combined with a need for good resolution then the problem becomes significant and a solution must be found.

Methods for Elimination of the Static Effect

In the preceeding paragraphs the effects of static build up and a means of assessing it have been described. As stated in the introduction a variety of methods have been tried in order to eliminate these unwanted effects (Moss, unpublished observations) including sprays, plate-dampening and earthing strips. Any improvements were small and temporary. In an attempt to find a solution to this problem we investigated a number of different options.

Initially several different aperture plates were tried as alternatives to the standard 20mm open aperture (std). These were a 10mm open (10mm), 5mm open (5mm), 20mm open with 3 longitudinal wires (W), 20mm Mylar-covered (M) and 20mm "foil" covered (F). Mylar is a very thin sheet of metal-coated plastic which is, unfortunately, too thick to allow weak β-particles through. This type of aperture cannot therefore be used to detect ^{3}H. The "foil" is a thin sheet of metal with numerous slits across its width giving the effect of many cross-wires. These last two apertures were provided by the manufacturer.

The instrument was calibrated for each different aperture before measurements were made. The cpm detected and the C/M ratios obtained with increasing analysis time for each aperture are shown in Figure 3.

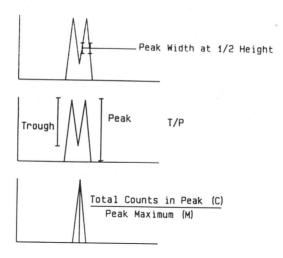

Fig. 2.   Methods of assessing instrumental (as opposed to chromatographic) resolution.

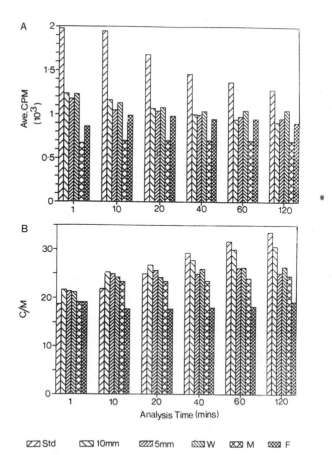

Fig. 3.   (A) CPM and (B) C/M values for each aperture with increasing analysis time.

We observed that narrowing the aperture gave more consistant results than the standard aperture but, as might be anticipated, with decreased sensitivity. The longitudinally wired aperture gave sensitivity and resolution equivalent to the narrowest open aperture. The "foil" covered aperture gave the best resolution and was more sensitive than the Mylar covered aperture but the efficiency was reduced to approximately 50% of that expected from an open detector in the absence of the static effect.

CONCLUSIONS

If the use of a linear analyzer with an unscreened detector is contemplated then it is important that the potential for a build up of static is investigated. If it is evident that such a build up is occurring then the extent to which it affects the results should be determined and, if necessary, steps taken to eliminate this as a source of error.

In our hands the "foil" gave the best overall solution and still permitted use of the instrument for ^3H. The Mylar film gave the best protection to the detector by excluding solvents, dust and other fine particulate material which might otherwise contaminate the detector but did not permit the detection of ^3H labelled compounds.

REFERENCE

1. H. Filthuth, Analytical and Chromatographic Techniques in Radiopharmaceutical Chemistry, D. H. Wieland, T. J. Mangner, M. Tobes, eds., Springer Verlag, New York, p. 79 (1985).

SORBENTS AND MODIFIERS

NEW SORBENTS FOR THIN-LAYER CHROMATOGRAPHY

W. Fischer, H. E. Hauck and W. Jost

E. Merck
P. O. box 4119
D-6100 Darmstadt, FRG

SUMMARY

The chromatographic and physical properties of surface-modified pre-coated supports for thin-layer chromatography are discussed. For reversed-phase supports substance Rf values decrease with the length of the alkyl chain and the degree of modification. Likewise, for a given solvent of constant composition the times required for development become longer. Owing to their pronounced hydrophobic nature reversed-phase supports which have been modified to the maximum extent can only be used with mobile phases having a water content not exceeding approximately 40%. This limitation does not apply, however, to reversed-phase supports having a defined low degree of surface modification.

Similarly, the hydrophilic aminopropyl and cyanopropyl modified plates do not impose any limitations to solvent composition. These medium-polar pre-coated layers can offer a wide range of interactions including ion exchange, adsorption, and hydrophobic interactions.

INTRODUCTION

The development of surface-modified sorbents and pre-coated layers has given thin-layer chromatography (TLC) new impetus, particularly in view of the reproducibility and the selectivities that can now be achieved. The growing number of publications on this topic bears witness to the increasing importance of modified supports in TLC[1-19].

The first and most important group of surface-modified TLC sorbents are the reversed-phase (RP) supports in which non-polar alkyl groups are chemically bonded to a silica gel skeleton. These hydrophobic sorbents eliminate the problems of poor reproducibility and partial elution of the liquid stationary phase, problems which were previously difficult to overcome but inherent in the use of impregnated TLC supports. Moreover, the introduction of chemically modified pre-coated RP plates enables the user for the first time to optimise phase systems for liquid column chromatography (in which approximately 80% of all separations are performed on RP phases), by applying TLC with chromatographically comparable support materials. This has led to considerable economies in terms both of time and cost.

139

The hydrophilic modified pre-coated plates which were subsequently
introduced also afford the same advantages of improved reproducibility and
outstanding stability against various solvent systems. Also, the surface-
bonded medium-polar functional groups of these hydrophilic modified supports afford new, specific selectivities.

EXPERIMENTAL

Various TLC and high performance (HP) TLC pre-coated plates of varying
alkyl chain lengths and degrees of modification were used as well as hydrophilic modified HPTLC cyanopropyl (CN) and aminopropyl (NH$_2$) pre-coated
plates (all from E. Merck, Darmstadt). Hamilton micro-syringes were used
to apply samples. Development was by the ascending method in normal
chambers without chamber saturation. Details of chromatographic conditions
are given in the captions to the figures. Chromatogram detection and
evaluation was accomplished with the aid of a TLC/HPTLC scanner from CAMAG,
Muttenz.

RESULTS AND DISCUSSION

Reversed-Phase Pre-Coated Layers

The chromatographic properties of reversed-phase pre-coated layers are
determined by the length of the alkyl chains chemically bonded to the
surface of the silica gel and by the degree of chemical modification. The
most popular RP modifications are of the RP-2, RP-8 and RP-18 type. The
numbers in the designation refer to the respective alkyl chain lengths,
except for the RP-2 modification, in which a dimethyl function is bound to
the surface.

In the RP modification series the hydrophobic character of the supports becomes more pronounced, for a similar degree of modification, as the
alkyl chain becomes longer. The retention of cholesterol serves as an
example to illustrate this property. Thus the Rf values for cholesterol on
RP-2, RP-8 and RP-18 HPTLC pre-coated plates are listed in Table 1. The
solvent composition was the same in each case (acetone/water 95/5 [v/v]).

As shown in Table 1 the Rf value for cholesterol decreases as the
stationary phase becomes more hydrophobic in character or, in other words,
substance retention increases in the same order.

Table 1. The Dependence of the Rf-Values of Cholesterol on the Alkyl
          Chain Length of RP Sorbents of Pre-Coated Plates

plates	:	HPTLC pre-coated plate RP-2 F 254s
		HPTLC pre-coated plate RP-8 F 254s
		HPTLC pre-coated plate RP-18 F 254s
eluent	:	acetone/water 95/5 (v/v)
migration distance	:	5cm
chamber	:	normal without chamber saturation

Type of plates	Rf-value of cholesterol
RP-2	0.86
RP-8	0.50
RP-18	0.14

For a constant alkyl chain length the hydrophobic character of an RP phase is determined by the respective degree of modification. This is of special importance in thin-layer chromatography, as the wettability of the stationary phase with highly polar solvents is determined by the hydrophobicity of the layer. Consequently, a maximally modified RP support can no longer be developed using highly aqueous solvents, since in this case the hydrophobic repulsive forces are stronger than the capillary forces moving the solvent through the support. The change in hydrophobicity of an RP support in TLC as a function of the degree of modification is of consequence not only for wettability (and thus also the flow characteristics) but also for determining substance retention.

As an illustration, Table 2 compares the HPTLC RP-18 precoated plate (an example of a maximally modified RP precoated support) with the HPTLC RP-18 W pre-coated plate (which represents an RP layer of a defined lower degree of modification and consequent lower hydrophobicity). For this purpose the retention of various polycyclic hydrocarbons is examined.

Thus the retention values for fluoroanthene, 3,4-benzofluoroanthene and indeno(1,2,3,c,d)pyrene (Table 2) show that, with a polar mobile phase, the hydrophobic interactions with the non-polar sample substance are much weaker on the HPTLC RP-18 W plate than on the maximally modified HPTLC RP-18 plate.

Conversely, the larger number of non-reacted silanol groups on the silica gel skeleton of the HPTLC RP-18 W plate can influence the retention of sample substances more intensely (especially when relatively non-polar solvent systems are used) than is the case with the highly modified HPTLC RP-18 layer. This is apparent in Figure 1, in which various lipophilic dyestuffs were developed on the two types of HPTLC RP-18 plate with toluene as solvent.

Owing to the considerably more pronounced silanol activity on the HPTLC RP-18 W plate, the dyes were much more strongly retained than on the maximally modified HPTLC RP-18 plate. When using RP plates with differing degrees of modification it is important to realise that there will be a significant span of selectivities and retention not only for the usual aqueous mobile phases but also in "Non Aqueous Reversed-Phase (NARP)" chromatography.

Table 2. The Dependence of the Rf-Values of Some Polycyclic Aromatic Hydrocarbons on the Degree of Modification of RP Pre-Coated Plates

plates	: HPTLC pre-coated plate RP-18 F 254s
	HPTLC pre-coated plate RP-18 W F 254s
eluent	: acetonitrile/water 90/10 (v/v)
migration distance	: 5 cm
chamber	: normal chamber without chamber saturation

| Type of plates | Rf-values of | | |
	Fluoroanthene	Benzo(k)fluoroanthene	Indeno(1,2,3-c,d)pyrene
RP-18	0.33	0.17	0.11
RP-18W	0.72	0.58	0.47

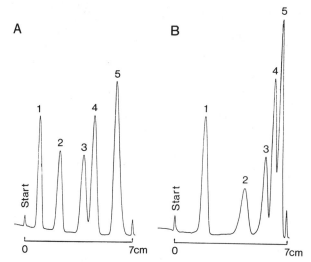

Fig. 1. Residual adsorption characteristics of HPTLC reversed-phase layers
- separation of lipophilic dyes. Plates: A. HPTLC pre-coated
plate RP-18 W F 254s, B. HPTLC pre-coated plate RP-18 F 254s.
Eluent: toluene. Migration distance: 5 cm. Chamber: normal chamber
without chamber saturation. Compounds: 1: Ceresred G, 2: Solvent
Violet 37, 3: Solvent Blue 104, 4: Violet in Ceresblack G, 5:
Ceresviolet BRN. (All 0.1%). Application volume: 200 nl.
Detection: in-situ evaluation with TLC/HPTLC scanner (Camag) UV
555 nm.

Chain lengths and the degree of chemical modification affect the
development time characteristics of pre-coated RP layers in addition to
their retention characteristics. Also, the mean particle size and the
particle size distribution of the silica gel support used have a not in-
considerable influence on the running characteristics of RP layers.

In Figure 2 the migration times for a methanol-water mixture (60:40
[v/v]) over a migration distance of 7cm as a function of the alkyl chain
length of two TLC RP pre-coated plates are compared. As is to be expected,
the TLC RP-18 plate, through its more pronounced hydrophobic character,
requires a longer development time than the corresponding RP-8 plate.

Since, in TLC, movement of solvent through the layer occurs exclusively through capillary forces, it is vital for the solvent to wet the
stationary phase completely. This requirement is no longer fulfilled,
however, when a highly modified RP layer is used with highly aqueous mobile
phases. In such cases only an RP layer with marked remanent hydrophilicity
can be used. Deliberately induced, reproducible remanent hydrophilicity is
achieved by a defined low degree of modification.

Thus Figure 3 compares the flow characteristics of a maximally modified HPTLC RP-18 plate with those of an HPTLC RP-18 W plate of defined low
modification. Acetone-water 70:30 [v/v] was used as mobile phase over a
migration distance of 5cm. The distinct differences in running times on
these two RP-18 plates are entirely attributable to the different degrees
of modification. As expected, the maximally modified HPTLC RP-18 plate has
a much longer running time. On account of its pronounced hydrophobicity,
this RP support can only be used with solvent systems having a water content not exceeding approximately 40% by volume. By contrast, the less

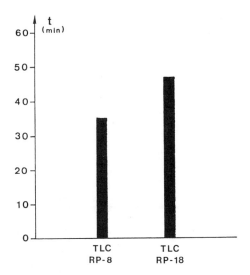

Fig. 2. The dependence of the migration time on the alkyl chain length of RP sorbents of precoated plates. Plates: TLC pre-coated RP-8 F 254s, TLC pre-coated plate RP-18 F 254s. Eluent: methanol/water 60/40 (v/v). Migration distance: 7 cm. Chamber: normal chamber without chamber saturation.

modified RP-18 W plate can be used without any restrictions as to solvent composition; indeed, it can even be developed using pure water.

As well as by the nature and degree of chemical modification the flow characteristics of RP layers are determined by the mean particle size and particle size distribution of the basic silica gels.

This is illustrated in Figure 4 which shows the development times for two solvent systems (acetone-water 20:80 and 40:60 [v/v]) on a TLC RP-18 plate and an HPTLC RP-18 W plate, the migration distance being 5cm in both cases. These two RP layers have identical alkyl chain lengths and are of similar hydrophobicity but differ, above all, in their mean particle size (TLC approx. 11-12 µm; HPTLC approx. 5-6 µm), with the HPTLC layer having a markedly narrower particle size distribution than the TLC layer. This means that although the migration distance and solvent composition are the same in both cases, the HPTLC layer needs longer development times. However, the smaller mean particle size of the HPTLC layers coupled with the narrower particle size distribution gives a denser packing, a smoother surface structure and superior chromatographic separation efficiency.

In RP chromatography the retention and separation of non-polar substances is attributable to hydrophobic interactions with the non-polar stationary phase. A typical example of the way in which the retention of sample substances increases with hydrophobicity is shown in the separation of fatty acid isatin methyl esters in Figure 5. It is also possible in RP chromatography to add ion-pair reagents to the solvent, for example, as a means of selectively retaining polar, charged substances. In the separation of various analgesic substances in Figure 6 adding tetramethylammonium bromide serves not only to influence the retention characteristics but also to compress the spots (See also Ruane and Wilson, this volume).

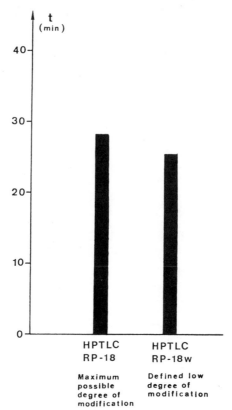

Fig. 3. Influence of degree of modification on the migration time of RP
pre-coated plates with identical mean particle sizes. Plates:
HPTLC pre-coated plate RP-18 F 254s, HPTLC pre-coated RP-18W F
254s. Eluent: acetone-water 70:30 (v/v). Migration distance:
5 cm. Chamber: normal chamber without chamber saturation.

Hydrophilic Modified Pre-Coated Layers

Leaving aside the non-polar modified RP layers discussed above, the
recently introduced hydrophilic modified pre-coated plates have also broadened the spectrum of selectivities available for TLC. The plates in
question are the HPTLC NH_2 pre-coated plate, in which γ-aminopropyl groups
are bonded to the surface of the silica gel skeleton, and the HPTLC CN
pre-coated plate with γ-cyanopropyl groups as functional groups. In terms
of polarity the two hydrophilic modifications can be classified as follows:

$$SiO_2 > NH_2 > CN > RP$$

Since the surface NH_2 and CN groups are of medium polarity, no wetting
problems are encountered with these plates, even at maximum degrees of
modification, and any solvent system can be used without restriction.

Through its functional group the NH_2 support can act as a weakly basic
ion exchanger and be used, for example, to separate charged substances.
The separation of various nucleotide building blocks, depicted in Figure 7,
occurs on the basis of differing charge numbers, with substances being more
strongly retained as their charge number increases.

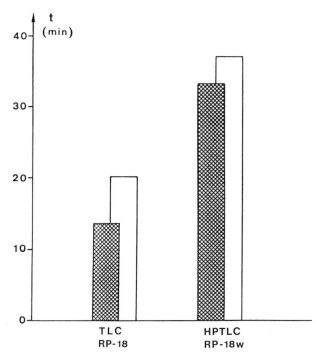

Fig. 4. Influence of particle size on the migration times of RP pre-coated
         plates with comparable degree of modification. Plates: TLC
         pre-coated plate RP-18 F 254s, HPTLC pre-coated plate RP-18W F
         254s. Eluent: acetone-water ▨▨ 20:80 (v/v), ▭ 40:60 (v/v).
         Migration distance: 5 cm. Chamber: normal chamber without chamber
         saturation.

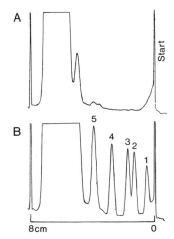

Fig. 5. Separation of fatty acids as isatin methyl esters. Derivat-
         isation: reaction of the fatty acids with 1-chloromethylisatin.
         Plate: HPTLC pre-coated plate RP-18 F 254s. Eluent: methanol-
         water 88:12 (v/v). Migration distance: 8 cm. Chamber: normal
         chamber without chamber saturation. Compounds: isatin esters of:
         1: Myristic acid, 2: Tridecanoic acid, 3: Lauric acid, 4: n-Capric
         acid, 5: Caprylic acid. Detection: in-situ evaluation with
         TLC/HPTLC scanner (Camag) UV 313 nm. Application of reaction
         mixture: A. chromatogram of reaction mixture without fatty acids,
         B. chromatogram of reaction mixture.

145

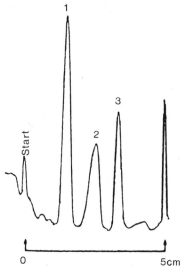

Fig. 6. Separation of ingredients in analgesics. Plate: HPTLC pre-coated
plate RP-18W F 254s. Eluent: methanol-water 30:70 (v/v) with
addition of 0.1 mol/1 TMABr. Migration distance: 5 cm. Chamber:
normal chamber without chamber saturation. Compounds: 1
Ethylmorphine hydrochloride (0.1%), 2 Scopolamine (3.0%), 3
Morphine hydrochloride (0.3%). Application volume: 300 nl.
Detection: in-situ evaluation with TLC/HPTLC scanner (Camag) UV
254 nm.

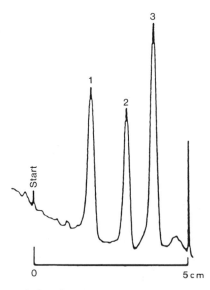

Fig. 7. Separation of nucleotide units. Plate: HPTLC pre-coated plate NH_2
F 254s. Eluent: methanol-water 90/10 (v/v) with addition of 0,2
mol/1 lithium chloride. Migration distance: 5 cm. Chamber:
normal chamber without chamber saturation. Compounds: 1:
[Adenylyl-(3'→5')]$_2$-adenosine, 2: Adenylyl-(3'→5')-adenosine,
3: Adenosine, (all 0.1%). Application volume: 200 nl. Detection:
in-situ evaluation with TLC/HPTLC scanner (Camag) UV 254 nm.

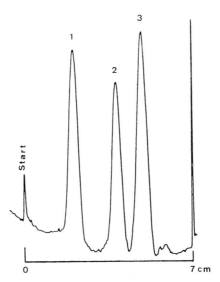

Fig. 8. Separation of oligo nucleotides. Plate: HPTLC pre-coated plate
NH₂ F 254s. Eluent: ethanol–water 10:90 (v/v) with addition of
0.1 mol/l lithium chloride. Migration distance: 7 cm. Chamber:
normal chamber without chamber saturation. Compounds: 1:
Adenylyl-(3'→5')-uridylyl-(3'→5')-guanosine, 2: [Adenylyl-
(3'→5')]₂-uridine, 3: [Adenylyl-(3'→5')]₂-cytidine, (all 0.1%).
Application volume: 200 nl. Detection: in-situ evaluation with
TLC/HPTLC scanner (Camag) UV 254 nm.

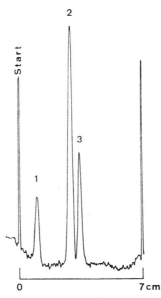

Fig. 9. Separation of estrone derivatives. Plate: HPTLC pre-coated plate
CN F 254s. Eluent: petroleum benzene (40–60°C)–acetone 80:20
(v/v). Migration distance: 7 cm. Chamber: normal chamber without
chamber saturation. Compounds: 1: Estriol, 2: Estradiol, 3:
Estrone, (all 0.1%). Application volume: 200 nl. Detection:
spray reagent: MnCl₂–sulfuric acid heating up to 120°C for 10 min.
UV 366 nm.

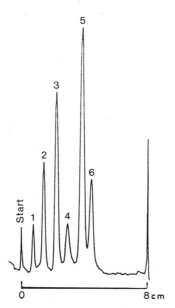

Fig. 10. Separation of DNP amino acids. Plate: HPTLC pre-coated plate CN
F 254s. Eluent: acetone-methanol-water 45:10:45 (v/v/v) with
addition of 0.1 mol/1 lithium chloride. Migration distance:
8 cm. Chamber: normal chamber without chamber saturation.
Compounds: 1: N,O-DNP-L-Tyrosine, 2: N,S-di-DNP-L-Cysteine,
3: N-DNP-L-Valine, 4: N-DNP-L-Proline, 5: N-DNP-L-Serine,
6: N-DNP-L-Asparagine, (all 0.2%). Application volume: 400 nl.
Detection: in-situ evaluation with TLC/HPTLC scanner (Camag) UV
254 nm.

Additionally, other retention mechanisms can be involved in retaining
sample substances on the NH_2 plate. For example, Figure 8 shows the separation of various oligonucleotides; the selectivity arises through differences in the hydrophobicity of the various nucleobases.

The CN modified layer can be used for both normal phase and reversed-phase chromatography, all according to the polarity of the solvent systems used.

The separation of estrogen derivatives in Figure 9 with petroleum benzene-acetone as solvent proceeds in a manner analogous to a normal-phase retention mechanism i.e. adsorption chromatography. In Figure 10, on the other hand, the separation of dinitrophenyl amino acids shows that the CN layer also exhibits the properties of an RP support.

CONCLUSION

The introduction of polar and non-polar surface modifications has considerably broadened the spectrum of selectivities achievable in thin-layer chromatography. The way has now also been opened for developing and optimising chromatographic conditions for HPLC by using comparable stationary phases in TLC.

148

REFERENCES

1. A. M. Siouffi, T. Wawrzynowics, J. Chromatogr., 186:563 (1979).
2. U. A. Th. Brinkman, G. de Vries, J.High.Resolut.Chromatogr.Chromatogr. Commun., 2:79 (1979).
3. H. Halpaap, K.-F. Krebs, H. E. Hauck, J.High Resolut.Chromatogr. Chromatogr.Commun., 3:215 (1980).
4. U. A. Th. Brinkman, G. de Vries, J.Chromatogr., 192:331 (1980).
5. D. Volkmann, J.High Resolut.Chromatogr.Chromatogr.Commun., 3:189 (1980).
6. G. A. Bens, W. Van den Bossche, P. de Moerloose, J.High Resolut. Chromatogr.Chromatogr.Commun., 3:433 (1980).
7. C. Gonnet, M. Marichy, J.Liq.Chromatogr., 3:1901 (1980).
8. K. Winsauer, W. Buchberger, Chromatographia 14:623 (1981).
9. A. M. Siouffi, G. Guiochon, J.Chromatogr., 209:441 (1981).
10. U. A. Th. Brinkman, G. de Vries, J.High Resolut.Chromatogr. Chromatogr.Commun., 5:476 (1982).
11. L. Lepri, P. G. Desideri, D. Heimler, J. Chromatogr., 235:411 (1982).
12. H. E. Hauck, W. Jost, Am.Lab., 15:72 (1983).
13. H. Heckers, F. W. Melcher, J.Chromatogr., 256:185 (1983).
14. R. Tomingas, Y. P. Grover, Fresenius Z. Anal.Chem., 315:515 (1983).
15. W. Jost, H. E. Hauck, J.Chromatogr., 261:235 (1983).
16. L. W. Doner, L. M. Biller, J.Chromatogr., 287:391 (1984).
17. G. Grassini-Strazza, I. Nicoletti, J.Chromatogr., 322:149 (1985).
18. M. Okamoto, F. Yamada, K. Adachi, J.High Resolut.Chromatogr. Chromatogr. Commun., 8:44 (1985).
19. W. Jost, H. E. Hauck, W. Fischer, Chromatographia 21:375 (1986)

THE IMPORTANCE OF THIN-LAYER CHROMATOGRAPHY AS A RAPID

METHOD FOR THE CONTROL OF OPTICAL PURITY

R. Rausch

Macherey-Nagel GmbH & Co. KG
P O Box 307
D-5160 Düren, W. Germany

SUMMARY

   The determination of the optical purity of natural or synthetic substances is a great challenge in analytical chemistry. As well as classical
methods for optical purity determination chromatographic methods are also
available and these are of high sensitivity. The main chromatographic
methods at the present time are gas chromatography and high-performance
liquid chromatography. However thin-layer chromatography also shows
potential for enantiomeric separations and the control of the optical
purity of certain types of compound.

INTRODUCTION

   In analytical chemistry enantiomeric separations are gaining more and
more interest. It is well known that the two isomers of a natural chiral
compound or a chiral synthetic drug can differ substantially in their
pharmacological activity depending on their absolute configuration. At
best one enantiomer is active, while the other is totally inactive. However, there are now examples of a number of drugs for which the effect of
one enantiomer can be disasterous. Some of these compounds are shown in
Table 1.

   To obtain pure enantiomers the function of preparative chemistry is to
develop stereoselective syntheses or, failing this, to accomplish the
separation of racemic mixtures at a preparative scale. In analytical
chemistry it is not only important to separate racemic mixtures but above
all to determine the concentration of the minor enantiomer in the excess of
the other, and determine and control the optical purity, which is characterized by the enantiomeric excess or "ee" value, defined as:

$$ee = \frac{a-b}{a+b} \qquad \begin{array}{l} a = \text{conc. of the predominant enantiomer} \\ b = \text{conc. of the minor enantiomer} \end{array}$$

or the % value ee x 100.

Table 1.

Compound type	Structure	Comment
Estrone		Estrogenic hormone effect(+)/inactive(−)
Barbiturates		Narcotic convulsions
Asparagine	$\overset{NH_2}{HO_2C\ CH\ CH_2\ CONH_2}$	Sweet (R)/bitter (S)
DOPA	HO—⟨ ⟩—CH$_2$CHCO$_2$H, NH$_2$	Treatment of Parkinsons disease (L)
Penicillamine	$\overset{Me\ NH_2}{HS\overset{\|}{C}\ CHCO_2H}$, Me	Antiarthritic (D)/ extremely toxic (L)
Thyroxine	HO—⟨ ⟩—O—⟨ ⟩—CH$_2$CHCO$_2$H, NH$_2$ (with I substituents)	Thyroid gland hormone (S) antihypercholesterinic (R)
Ethambutol	CH$_3$CH$_2$CHNHCH$_2$CH$_2$NHCH, CH$_2$OH ... CH$_2$OH, CH$_2$CH$_3$	Tuberculostatic (SS)/ blindness (RR)
Thalidomide		Sleep inducing (R)/ teratogenic (S)

152

METHODS FOR THE DETERMINATION OF OPTICAL PURITY

In order to determine the enantiomeric composition of mixtures of isomers the following methods are used: chiroptical methods, in particular polarimetry, NMR-spectroscopy and the chromatographic methods.

a) Polarimetry

Polarimetry is the most popular method for evaluating the ee value by measuring the rotation α of plane polarized light at a specific wavelength. Although this method is a relatively simple procedure, the correct determination of an enantiomeric composition is limited by some points. Some of these limitations are as follows, for example the maximum optical rotation of the pure enantiomer must be known with certainty, large sample sizes are required, the result depends on temperature, solvent and traces of optically active or inactive impurities. It is also important to ensure that sample preparation for analysis does not accidentally result in the enrichment of one or other of the enantiomers in the mixture. Provided that all these points are fulfilled, in most cases, the accuracy is between 2-3%. This means that for the control of optical purity an ee value of 96% is the best result that can be obtained.

b) Nuclear Magnetic Resonance Spectroscopy (NMR)

Another method frequently used to determine the enantiomeric composition of a substance is NMR spectroscopy, especially with the use of chiral lanthanide shift reagents, e.g. Eu-camphor complexes.

Such determinations are based on the diastereomeric association between a chiral organic substrate and a pure optical active lanthanide shift reagent. If the substrate is able to coordinate with the lanthanide ion, a chemical shift is induced. The result is one shifted signal if the enantiomer is pure or two shifted signals if it is a mixture. The proton integrals allow the enantiomeric ratio to be calculated. Usually, if only one peak is observed, the concentration of the minor antipode is less than 1.5%, which means that NMR methods can provide ee values of about 97%.

In practice, solubility problems may restrict the use of the technique. Traces of water or acidic impurities must also be avoided, and careful purification of the solvents and the substrate is recommended.

By using NMR methods the enantiomeric composition of amines, amides, alcohols, diols, aldehydes, esters, ethers, sulfoxides, phosphine oxides and some natural products have been determined.

c) Chromatographic Methods

As described below gas chromatography[1-5], high-performance liquid chromatography[6-12] as well as thin-layer chromatography[13-18] are all used to determine enantiomeric composition.

Gas Chromatography (GC)

GC has been used to resolve enantiomers for more than 20 years. In the case of the low molecular weight phases such as amino acids, dipeptides and tripeptides, disadvantages were their high melting point and bleeding of the phase at higher temperatures. Better results were obtained with diamide phases, but the major breakthrough was the synthesis of optically active polysiloxane stationary phases, which can be used between 30°C and 230°C.

The only phase which is commercially available is Chirasil-Val (D- or
L-form), the diamide of valine, immobilized on a polysiloxane. The separation mechanism is based on hydrogen-bonding effects. The Chirasil-Val
phase can be used for substances such as amino acids, amino alcohols,
amines, sugars, hydroxy acids, ketones and diketones. Nevertheless most of
them have to be derivatized, one of the disadvantages of the GC method. Of
course there are a great number of compounds such as alcohols, ketones,
epoxides, oxiranes and olefins which can be separated without derivatisation. However, despite this limitation GC as an analytical tool allows
the sensitive determination of the optical purity, and trace levels of the
minor enantiomer can be observed despite an excess of the major one. This
high sensitivity (on Chirasil-Val WCOT columns) enables enantiomeric
impurities of 0.1%, (an ee value of 99.8%) to be determined. Additionally
it is possible to analyze the enantiomeric composition of a complex mixture
simultaneously with excellent accuracy.

Another class of GC phase for enantiomeric separations, the chiral
metal chelates, are likely to become increasingly more important[19-23].

High Performance Liquid Chromatography (HPLC)

In HPLC the variety of different phases for optical resolution is much
greater than in GC, and many of these phase are commercially available[24].
According to the separation mechanism used one must distinguish between
ligand-exchange phases, affinity phases, helical polymer phases, cavity
phases and "brush-type" phases. There is currently a rapidly increasing
number of reports of applications for HPLC both with and without derivatisation in this area. Accuracy and sensitivity seem to be similar to the GC
methods.

Thin Layer Chromatography (TLC)

Relatively few publications currently exist concerning enantiomeric
separations by TLC[13-18].

On cyclodextrin some derivatized amino acids have been separated into
their enantiomers. Reversed-phase (RP) plates coated with a chiral selector and copper or a selector and copper in the eluent also allows separations of some amino acids. But the substances had to be derivatized and
the procedure of pretreatment of the plates was complicated. A direct
resolution of amino acids is possible on microcrystalline cellulose plates,
but the developing conditions are less than ideal. Thus the migration time
was 12 hours and the temperature 0°C. A "brush-type" phase succeeded in
only one separation of optical antipodes.

All these plates had the disadvantages of a long developing time, the
need for the substrate to be derivatized, poor resolution or complex experimental procedures. Additionally they are not commercially available.
Recently TLC plates, based on ligand exchange, were developed by Günther
and coworkers[25] and since 1985 this plate has been commercially available
as the Chiralplate[26].

The use of these plates, on which a great number of compounds have now
been separated[27-37] is described below.

Characterization of the Layer

The basic phase is a special modified RP-18 silica gel, which is first
loaded with Cu^{2+} by dipping in a aqueous/methanolic Cu(II) acetate solution
(0.25%). After drying a second dipping in a solution of a chiral selector
(Figure 1) follows:

154

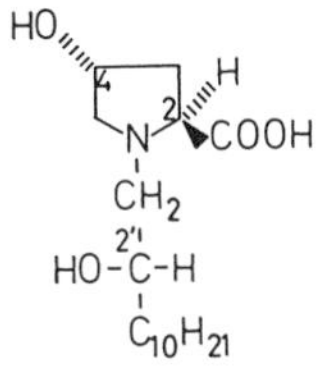

Fig. 1. Chiral TLC selector: (2S,4R,2'RS)-4-Hydroxy-1-(2-hydroxydodecyl) proline.

After dipping in the selector (0.8% in methanol) the plate is dried once again and it is ready to use.

Separation Mechanism

The separation mechanism is based on ligand exchange, it means the formation of diastereomeric complexes between the central Cu^{2+} ion, the chiral selector and the substrate. Enantiomeric resolution is possible, if the antipodes of a chiral substrate form complexes of different stability. This requirement, complex formation, is the only restriction for the use of the Chiralplate.

Separation Conditions

In practice 2μl of a 1% solution of the underivatised recemates (generally amino acids or related compounds) in methanol or methanol water are spotted on to the freshly activated layer. For many applications eluents composed of methanol-water-acetonitrile, (50:50:200, v/v/v, for eluent A, 50:50:30, v/v/v, for eluent B) with chamber saturation are suitable. For a migration distance between 12 and 14cm, the migration time is 25 minutes for eluent A and 60 to 70 minutes for eluent B. After drying the plate the spots are visualized using 0.1% ninhydrin spray reagent and heating at between 105 to 110°C for 5 minutes.

Examples

According to the separation mechanism the following substance classes form suitable complexes and are separated into individual enantiomers on the chiralplate.

- amino acids
- halogenated amino acids
- N-methylated amino acids
- N-formylated amino acids
- α-alkyl amino acids
- lactones
- dipeptides
- thiazolidine derivatives.

An example for the separation of amino acids is given in Figure 2, in Table 2 the R_F values and the eluents used are listed.

Normally all these compounds are chromatographed underivatised. Derivatisation is only necessary if a SH-group is contained in the molecule. In this case the formation of a thiazolidine ring with formaldehyde enables the application of the crude, unpurified product. This simple procedure was only necessary in two cases, the amino acids cysteine and penicillamine, but for about 100 compounds no derivatisation has proved necessary.

155

Table 2. Enantiomeric Separations on CHIRALPLATE

Racemates	R_F value (configuration)				Eluent[a]
Alanine derivatives					
D-Alanine-L-Phenylalanine	0.59				B
L-Alanine-D-Phenylalanine	0.65				B
3-Chloroalanine	0.57		0.64		A
3-Cyclopentylalanine	0.46		0.56		A
(1-Naphthyl)alanine	0.49	(D)	0.46	(L)	A
(2-Naphthyl)alanine	0.44	(D)	0.59	(L)	A
2-Amino butyric acid	0.48		0.52		A
3-Amino-3,5,5-trimethylbutyrolactone·HCl	0.50		0.59		A
Aspartic acid	0.50	(D)	0.55	(L)	A
Cysteine (derivatized)[b]	0.59	(D)	0.69	(L)	A
S-(2-Chlorobenzyl)-cysteine	0.45		0.58		A
S-(3-Thiabutyl)-cysteine	0.53		0.64		A
S-(2-Thiapropyl)-cysteine	0.53		0.64		A
Dopa (3,4-Dihydroxyphenylalanine)	0.47	(L)	0.58	(D)	B
α-Methyldopa	0.46	(L)	0.66	(D)	B
Ethionine	0.52	(D)	0.59	(L)	A
Ethioninesulfon	0.55		0.59		A
Glutamic acid	0.54	(D)	0.59	(L)	A
Glutamine	0.41	(L)	0.55	(D)	A
Glycine derivatives					
2-Cyclopentylglycine	0.43		0.50		A
Glycyl-Isoleucine	0.54	(L)	0.61	(D)	B
Glycyl-Leucine	0.53	(L)	0.60	(D)	B
Glycyl-Phenylalanine	0.57	(L)	0.63	(D)	B
Glycyl-Tryptophan	0.48	(L)	0.55	(D)	B
Glycyl-Valine	0.58	(L)	0.62	(D)	B
2-(1-Methylcyclopropyl)-glycine	0.49		0.57		A
2-Phenylglycine	0.57		0.67		A
Leucine derivatives	0.51	(D)	0.61	(L)	C
D-Leucine-L-Leucine	0.48				B
L-Leucine-D-Leucine	0.57				B
allo-Isoleucine	0.51	(D)	0.61	(L)	A
Isoleucine	0.47	(D)	0.58	(L)	A
Norleucine	0.53	(D)	0.62	(L)	A
N-Formyl-tert.-leucine	0.48	(+)	0.61	(−)	A
N-Methylleucine	0.49	(L)	0.57	(D)	A
tert.-Leucine	0.40	(D)	0.51	(L)	A
Methionine derivatives	0.54	(D)	0.59	(L)	A
D-Methionine-L-Methionine	0.64				B
L-Methionine-D-Methionine	0.71				B
Methioninesulfon	0.62	(D)	0.66	(L)	A
α-Methylmethionine	0.56	(D)	0.64	(L)	A
Selenomethionine	0.53	(D)	0.61	(L)	A

Table 2. (continued)

Racemates	R_F value (configuration)				Eluent[a]
Penicillamine (derivatized)[b]	0.48	(D)	0.62	(L)	A
Phenylalanine	0.49	(D)	0.59	(L)	A
4-Aminiphenylalanine	0.33		0.47		A
4-Bromophenylalanine	0.44		0.58		A
4-Chlorophenylalanine	0.46		0.59		A
2-Fluorophenylalanine	0.55		0.59		A
Homophenylalanine	0.49	(D)	0.58	(L)	A
4-Iodophenylalanine	0.45	(D)	0.61	(L)	A
4-Methoxyphenylalanine	0.52		0.64		A
α-Methylphenylalanine	0.53	(L)	0.66	(D)	A
N-Methylphenylalanine	0.50	(D)	0.61	(L)	A
4-Nitrophenylalanine	0.52		0.61		A
N,N-Dimethylphenylalanine	0.55	(D)	0.61	(L)	B
Proline	0.41	(D)	0.47	(L)	A
allo-4-Hydroxyproline	0.41	(L)	0.59	(D)	A
Serine					
O-Benzylserine	0.54	(D)	0.64	(L)	A
α-Methylserine	0.56	(L)	0.67	(D)	A
Thyroxine	0.39	(D)	0.49	(L)	A
Tryptophan	0.51	(D)	0.61	(L)	A
5-Bromotryptophan	0.46		0.58	(A)	A
N-Carbamyl-tryptophan	0.44	(L)	0.55	(D)	D
5-Methoxytryptophan	0.55		0.66		A
4-Methyltryptophan	0.50		0.58		A
5-Methyltryptophan	0.52		0.63		A
6-Methyltryptophan	0.52		0.64		A
7-Methyltryptophan	0.51		0.64		A
Tyrosine	0.58	(D)	0.66	(L)	A
O-Benzyltyrosine	0.48	(D)	0.64	(L)	A
3-Fluorotyrosine	0.64		0.71		A
α-Methyltyrosine	0.63	(D)	0.70	(L)	A
N-Methyl-m-tyrosine	0.36		0.52		B
Valine	0.54	(D)	0.62	(L)	A
N-Methylvaline	0.65	(L)	0.70	(D)	B
Norvaline	0.49	(D)	0.56	(L)	A

a) Eluents:
  A   Methanol/water/acetonitrile, 50/50/200 (v/v/v)
  B   Methanol/water/acetonitrile, 50/50/30 (v/v/v)
  C   Methanol/water, 10/80 (v/v)
  D   1 mM cupric acetate, 5% methanol (pH 5.8), 16°C, 4 hours,
      detection with Ehrlich's reagent[38]

b) derivatized with formaldehyde to thiazolidine derivative

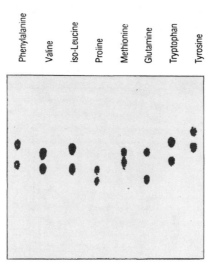

Fig. 2.   Enantiomeric separations of amino acids on Chiralplate.
Separation conditions see text.

Unfortunately some amino acids or bifunctional amino acids are not
separated on these plates.   It seems some functional groups are important
in the final conformation.   For example serine is not resolved in either
eluent A or B, but α-methylserine is separated.   The reason for this may be
that the additional methyl group interacts with the RP groups of the
layer[40].

Quantification and Control of Optical Purity

The quantification of the enantiomeric composition is possible with a
densitometer (Figure 3) and this is illustrated for D,L-tyrosine and D,L-
phenylalanine in Figure 3.

After visualization with ninhydrin the spots were detected at 520nm
(Shimadzu Dual-Wavelength TLC Scanner CS-930) with good reproducability.
Slightly better resolution and accuracy can be achieved with linear application of the racemates as a streak rather than a spot.   But certainly the
accuracy of the method is not as good as either GC or HPLC.

As well as quantification as described above the control of the optical purity of a substance requires the determination of trace levels of
one enantiomer in an excess of the other.   The results with a TLC Scanner
(conditions as above) are demonstrated in Figure 4.

On the left side the chromatogram of a pure standard of D-tyrosine is
shown and next to it the scan of a sample containing 0.1% L-tyrosine in
99.9% D-tyrosine, i.e. under these conditions an ee value of 99.8% may be
determined.   The right side shows the so-called "pure" L-enantiomer con-
taminated with a small amount of the D-enantiomer and the same separation
after the addition of 0.1% D-tyrosine.   Of course due to the presence of
some D-tyrosine in the "pure" L-tyrosine this final concentration obtained
for the D-isomer was higher than 0.1%.

Using only the unaided eye between 0.25 and 0.5% of the minor enantiomer can be detected.   All of these results were obtained with "normal"
quantities loaded onto the plate.   Overloading may give a higher sensitivity for the enantiomer with the higher R_F value.

158

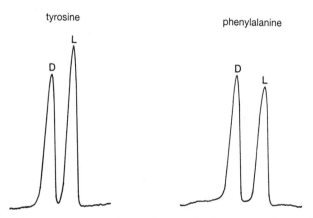

tyrosine

phenylalanine

Fig. 3. Enantiomeric separation of racemic D,L-tyrosine and
D,L-phenylalanine on Chiralplate detection with a densitometer
at 520 nm after visualization with ninhydrin.

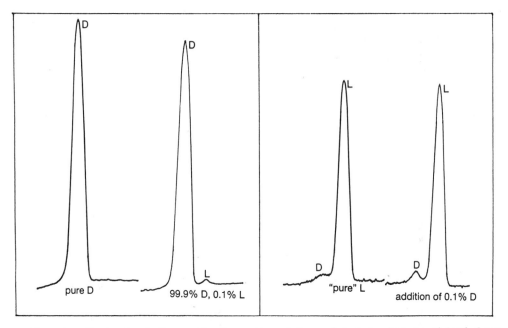

Fig. 4. Control of the optical purity of D- and L-tyrosine on Chiralplate.

Comparison of GC Versus TLC

Under normal circumstances GC separations are much more sensitive and
accurate than TLC separations. However, in this case we have a similar
sensitivity with ee values of about 99.8%.

With regard to ease of use the TLC method has some obvious advantages.
For example, for GC analysis there is the requirement for derivatisation in
order to make the amino acids volatile. Additionally any SH-groups have to
be reduced with Raney-nickel. These procedures are time consuming and in
addition racemisation may occur. Furthermore crude products from syntheses
or solutions of pharmaceutical preparations such as capsules or tablets
have to be removed before analysis. TLC with the Chiral-plate allows the

159

application of such crude mixtures without the need for prior purification. The TLC method is not only fast and simple but in comparison to GC also inexpensive.

However GC does allow the separation of a mixture of several enantiomers simultaneously, and is more versatile, whereas the Chiralplate is restricted to substances which can be separated by ligand exchange. This is a relatively small group – but includes some very important compounds. In particular the amino acids are building blocks for biologically active peptides, pure enantiomers are required for the synthesis of antibiotics, a low calorie sweetener, some insecticides and other pharmaceuticals such as dopa, methyldopa, penicillamine and thyroxine. D-phenylalanine has analgesic properties and might one day replace acetylsalicylic acid[39].

CONCLUSION

Currently one of the most demanding analytical problems, of ever increasing importance, is the determination of the enantiomeric composition of optically active compounds, particularly the control of the optical purity. Doubtless the most universal technique is polarimetry. But this method is not sensitive enough for the determination of trace levels of one antipode. Chromatographic methods such as GC and HPLC are much more sensitive, but time consuming, expensive and currently still restricted to certain substance classes. The TLC method using the Chiralplate is more restricted even than GC or HPLC to substances which can be separated by ligand exchange chromatography, however, where the method does work, it is elegant, fast, inexpensive and also very sensitive.

REFERENCES

1. E. Bayer, Z.Naturforsch, B38:1281 (1983).
2. B. Koppenhoefer and E. Bayer, Chromatographia 19:123 (1984).
3. B. Koppenhoefer and E. Bayer, J.Chromatogr.,Library 32:1 (1985).
4. H. Frank, W. Woiwode, G. Nicholson, and E. Bayer, Liebigs Ann.Chem., 354 (1981).
5. W. A. König, E. Steinbach, and K. Ernst, Angew.Chem. 96:516 (1984).
6. G. Blaschke and H. Markgraf, Arch.Pharm.(Weinheim) 317:465 (1984).
7. I. W. Wainer and Th. D. Doyle, Liq.Chromatogr. 2:88 (1984).
8. E. Busker and J. Martens, Z.Anal.Chem. 319:907 (1984).
9. E. Küsters and D. Giron, J.High Res.Chromatogr.Chromatogr.Commun.
10. D. Johns, Int.Lab. 17:66 (1987).
11. S. Allenmark, J.Biochem.Biophys.Methods 9:1 (1984).
12. B. Bomgren and S. Allenmark, J.Liq.Chromatogr. 9:667 (1986).
13. I. W. Wainer, C. A. Brunner and Th.D. Doyle, J.Chromatogr. 264:154 (1983).
14. S. Weinstein, Tetrahedron Lett. 25:985 (1984).
15. N. Grinberg and S. Weinstein, J.Chromatogr. 303:251 (1984).
16. R. Marchelli, R. Virgili, E. Armani and A. Dossena, J.Chromatogr. 355:354 (1986).
17. A. Alak and D. W. Armstrong, Anal.Chem. 58:582 (1986).
18. S. Yuasa, A. Shimada, M. Isoyama, T. Fukuhara and M. Hoh, Chromatographia 21:79 (1986).
19. V. Schurig and W. Bürkle, J.Am.Chem.Soc. 104:7573 (1982).
20. V. Schurig and R. Weber, Angew.Chem. 95:797 (1983).
21. V. Schurig and R. Weber, J.Chromatogr. 217:51 (1981).
22. V. Schurig and R. Weber, J.Chromatogr. 284:321 (1984).
23. V. Schurig, U. Leyrer and R. Weber, J.High Res.Chromatogr.,Chromatogr. Commun. 8:459 (1985).
24. R. Däppen, H. Arm, and V. R. Meyer, J.Chromatogr. 373:1 (1986).

25. K. Günther, J. Martens and M. Schickedanz, Angew.Chem.Int.Ed.Engl., 23:506 (1984).
26. Chiralplate is a product of Macherey-Nagel GmbH & Co. KG, P.O. Box 307, D-5160 Düren.
27. K. Günther, J. Martens and M. Schickedanz, Naturwissenschaften 72:149 (1985).
28. K. Günther and R. Rausch, Proceedings of the 3rd International Symposium on Instrumental HPTLC, Würzburg, 1985, Institute for Chromatography, Bad Dürkheim, 469 (1985).
29. U.A. Th. Brinkman and D. Kamminga, J.Chromatogr., 330:375 (1985).
30. K. Günther, J. Martens and M. Schickedanz, Z.Anal.Chem., 322:513 (1985).
31. K. Günther, J. Martens and M. Schickedanz, Angew.Chem. 98:284 (1986). Angew.Chem.Int.Ed.Engl., 25:278 (1986).
32. K. Günther, J. Martens and M. Schickedanz, Arch.Pharm.(Weinheim), 319:461 (1986).
33. K. Günther, J. Martens and M. Schickedanz, Arch.Pharm.(Weinheim) 319:572 (1986).
34. K. Günther, M. Schickedanz, K. Drauz, and J. Martens, Z.Anal.Chem., 325:298 (1986).
35. K. Günther, GIT Suppl. 3:6 (1986).
36. C. Syldatk, D. Cotoras, A. Möller and F. Wagner, Biotech-Forum 3:9 (1986).
37. B. K. Vriesema, W. ten Hoeve, H. Wynberg, and R. M. Kellogg, Tetrahedron Lett., 26:2045 (1986).
38. L. K. Gont and S. K. Neuendorf, Incell Corporation, 1600 W. Cornell, Milwaukee, Wisconsin 53211 (USA), personal communication.
39. E. M. Mejer, W. H. J. Boesten, H. E. Schoemaker, and J. A. M. van Balken, "Biocatalysts in Organic Syntheses," Elsevier Science Publishers, B.V., Amsterdam, p. 1335 (1985).
40. V. A. Davankov, A. S. Bochkov and A. A. Kurganov, Chromatographia 13:677 (1980).

NORMAL AND REVERSED-PHASE ION-PAIR THIN-LAYER CHROMATOGRAPHY

WITH BIFUNCTIONAL (BOLAFORM) REAGENTS

R. J. Ruane and I. D. Wilson

Drug Metabolism Section, Safety of Medicines Department
Imperial Chemical Industries PLC, Mereside
Alderley Park, Macclesfield, Cheshire SK10 4TG

SUMMARY

The properties of three bisquaternary ammonium (bolaform) ion-pair reagents for ion-pair thin-layer chromatography have been investigated using a total of 8 organic acids as model compounds. The reagents used were 1,3-bis(trimethylammonium), 1,3-bis(triethylammonium) and 1,3-bis-(tripropylammonium)propane (all as dibromide salts). Reversed-phase chromatography was performed on silica gel, C_{18} bonded silica gel and paraffin coated silica gel with methanol-water based solvents. For normal-phase chromatography on silica gel dichloromethane-methanol mixtures were used. All three bolaform compounds behaved as ion-pair reagents, however, the properties of the bistripropyl compound were significantly different from those of the bistrimethyl and bistriethyl reagents. A possible reason for the observed differences, involving the interaction of the compounds with free silanol groups, is discussed.

INTRODUCTION

In the course of studies on the use of ion-pair (IP) reagents for reversed-phase thin-layer-chromatography (RP-TLC)[1-4] we have begun to investigate the properties of a number of bifunctional (bolaform) bis-quaternary ammonium compounds[3,4]. These bolaform ion-pair reagents appeared to have a number of useful and interesting properties, in particular it was possible to use them with a wider range of solvent compositions than "conventional" IP-reagents such as tetra-n-butylammonium bromide, and in both normal and reversed-phase modes of chromatography. In these initial experiments two compounds, 1,3 bis(trimethylammonium)propane and 1,12-bis(trimethylammonium)dodecane, were used and we noted that, despite large differences in molecular weight and the length of the "spacer" connecting the two quaternary ammonium groups, their properties were similar[4]. This behavior contrasts markedly with the effects observed when chain length was varied with more conventional mono-quaternary ammonium compounds[3]. For example an increase in chain length from C6 in (trimethylammonium)hexane bromide to C_{14} in cetyltrimethylammonium bromide (cetrimide), resulted not unexpectedly in a large decrease in the R_F of a range of aromatic acids.

Another unusual feature of IP-TLC with bolaform reagents was that, as the content of methanol in the solvent was increased to 80% and above, a reduction rather than an increase in R_F was obtained together with a reversal in the migration order of the test compounds(3,4).

In order to obtain a better understanding of the behavior of these bolaform IP-reagents, and also to determine the effect of structural modification on their properties, we have now studied two further compounds, 1,3-bis(triethylammonium) and 1,3-bis(tripropylammonium)propane (both as bromide salts). These new reagents were compared with the previously studied 1,3-bis(trimethylammonium)propane (bromide salt). Both normal and reversed-phase chromatography of eight aromatic acids using these three reagents has been investigated.

EXPERIMENTAL

Synthesis of Ion-Pair Reagents

The reagent 1,3-bis(trimethylammonium)propane dibromide was synthesised as described previously[4]. The synthesis of 1,3-bis(triethylammonium)propane dibromide was accomplished by mixing 1,3-dibromopropane (Aldrich Chemicals UK) with an excess of triethylamine (Rathburn, Scotland) and leaving the mixture overnight at room temperature. The reaction mixture was then diluted with n-hexane (BDH, Dorset, UK) and cooled to 0°C. This resulted in the crystallisation of the product (1,3 bis(triethylammonium)propane dibromide) which was filtered, washed with fresh hexane and freeze dried overnight.

The 1,3-bis(tripropylammonium)propane dibromide reagent was synthesised by mixing tripropylamine (BDH, Dorset, UK) and 1,3 dibromopropane in equimolar proportions then refluxing for 2 hours. The resulting oil was extracted with hexane to remove unreacted starting material. The product was triturated with diethyl ether and then dissolved in hot ethyl acetate. On cooling to 0°C 1,3 bis(tripropylammonium)propane dibromide crystallised out. The product was washed with cold ethyl acetate and freeze dried overnight to remove residual solvent.

It should be noted that both 1,3 bis(triethylammonium)propane dibromide and 1,3 bis(tripropylammonium)propane were hygroscopic. These reagents were therefore stored in a dessicator until used.

Chemicals

The test acids 2,4-dihydroxybenzoic acid, 1; 2,6-dihydroxybenzoic acid, 2; gentistic acid, 3; and salicylic acid, 4; were obtained from BDH Ltd (Poole, UK), benzoic acid, 5; p-chlorobenzoic acid, 6; O-nitrobenzoic acid, 7; and hydroxyhippuric acid, 8; were obtained from Sigma (Poole, UK).

Solvents were of HPLC grade and were obtained from Fisons (Loughborough, UK). All chemical and solvents were used as received.

Preparation of TLC plates

Silica gel and C_{18} bonded silica gel glass backed TLC plates (E Merck) 20 x 10cm incorporating a fluorescent indicator (254 mm) were obtained from BDH Ltd (Poole, UK). The plates were cut to size before use (5 x 10 cm) and then coated with an ion-pair reagent by dipping in a 0.1 M solution of the reagents in methanol. Similarly, paraffin-impregnated ion-pair coated plates were prepared by dipping silica gel TLC plates in 0.1 M solutions of ion-pair reagent dissolved in a mixture of methanol-dichloromethane containing 7.5% (v/v) paraffin BP (Hills Pharmaceuticals, Burnley, UK).

Chromatography

Ascending chromatography was performed in glass TLC tanks 10 x 10 x 5 cm using solvent systems of methanol-water for reversed-phase separations and dichloromethane-methanol for normal-phase chromatography. Compounds were visualized after chromatography by fluorescence quenching at 254 nm.

RESULTS

TLC on C_{18} Bonded RP-TLC Plates

Chromatography of any of the eight test acids on C_{18} bonded TLC plates in the absence of ion-pair reagent produced, for most solvent compositions, a streak extending from the origin to the solvent front. Only with a solvent containing 80% of methanol was an improvement in spot shape seen, whilst with 100% methanol all compounds ran at the solvent front. Coating the plates with any one of the three bolaform IP-reagents resulted in an immediate improvement in chromatography with good spot shape and R_F values increasing in a regular manner with increasing methanol content. Overall the bistripropyl reagent appeared to give the best spot shape with the bistrimethyl giving the worst. At 100% methanol all the compounds ran just below the solvent front, irrespective of the IP reagent used.

Typical results for representative compounds are illustrated in Figure 1, whilst the results for all eight compounds are to be found in Table 1.

These results show that, apart from the minor differences in spot shape mentioned above, there do not appear to be large differences in the properties of the three ion pair reagents on C_{18} bonded silica gel. Certainly there is no obvious trend to be seen as the size of the substituents surrounding the quaternised nitrogen are increased. For example for compound 1 an R_F value of 0.25 is obtained for the bistrimethyl reagent, 0.12 for the bistriethyl and 0.29 for the bistripropyl reagent respectively. Intuitively a reduction in R_F with increasing chain length might have been expected but this is clearly not the case.

TLC on Paraffin Coated Silica Gel TLC Plates

On control plates, coated only with paraffin, all the test acids migrated at, or near, the solvent front irrespective of solvent composition. When simultaneously coated with any one of the three ion-pair reagents a significant reduction in R_F was observed. However, the result of gradually increasing the eluotropic strength of the solvent were different to those obtained on the C_{18}-bonded plates (where a regular increase in the R_F of the test acids had been observed). Thus, with solvents containing between 0 to 40 or 60% of methanol (the exact proportion depending upon the reagent) a steady increase in R_F was noted with increasing methanol content. However, in the cases of both the bistrimethyl and bistriethyl reagents higher concentrations of methanol in the mobile phase resulted in a significant decrease in R_F. This result is consistent with our previous observations when the properties of the bistrimethyl reagents were investigated[3,4]. On paraffin coated silica gel the bistripropyl reagent gave very poor results with, for the majority of the compounds tested, badly distorted spots running close to the solvent front. These spots were generally so misshapen that, with solvents containing above 40% methanol, accurate R_F values could not be determined. In fact results were only obtained over the whole range of solvent compositions for compound 2

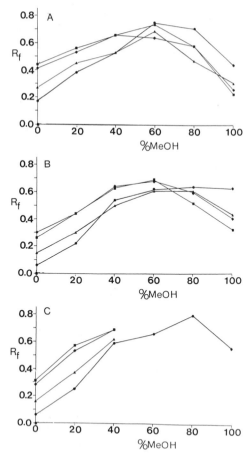

Fig. 1.   IP–RP–TLC on C_{18} bonded silica gel of 2,4–dihydroxybenzoic acid
(■), 2,6–dihydroxybenzoic acid (●), gentistic acid (♦) and
salicylic acid (▲). Methanol–water solvent systems were used with
plates impregnated with either 1,3–bistrimethyl (A); 1,3–
bistriethyl (B), or 1,3–bistripropylammonium (C) ion–pair
reagents.

(2,6–dihydroxybenzoic acid). Interestingly this compound, having increased
in R_F as solvent strength was increased from 0 to 60% methanol, then showed
a decrease in R_F from 0.8 at 80% to 0.56 at 100% methanol, i.e. behavior –
typical of the other bolaform reagents.

In general the R_F values obtained for the bistriethyl reagent coated
plates were roughly half those of the bistrimethyl reagent coated plates
with 100% water as solvent. The R_F values for the bistripropyl reagent,
for the same solvent were similar to those obtained for the bistrimethyl
compound. As the eluotropic strength of the solvent was increased these
differentials were gradually lost until by 40% methanol the R_F values
produced by all three reagents were broadly similar. The relationship
between R_F and solvent composition for a number of representative compounds
is illustrated in Figure 2, whilst results for all of the compounds are
given in Table 2.

Table 1. Variation of R with Solvent Composition of 8 Organic Acids for C_{18} bonded Silica Gel on IP-TLC with 1,3-bistrimethyl; 1,3-bistriethyl and 1,3-bistripropylammonium IP-reagents

% Methanol	0	20	40	60	80	100
Compound*			R_F			
1,3-bis(trimethylammonium)propane dibromide						
1	0.0	0.08	0.25	0.45	0.70	SF
2	0.0	0.04	0.20	0.41	0.67	SF
3	0.0	0.10	0.27	0.45	0.72	SF
4	0.0	0.07	0.16	0.35	0.67	SF
5	0.0	0.08	0.13	0.29	0.58	SF
6	0.0	0.0	0.05	0.16	0.17	SF
7	0.0	0.08	0.20	0.47	0.72	SF
8	0.0	0.04	0.16	0.37	0.63	SF
1,3-bis(triethylammonium)propane dibromide						
1	0.0	0.05	0.12	0.30	0.52	SF
2	0.0	0.0	0.09	0.25	0.45	SF
3	0.0	0.07	0.18	0.32	0.53	SF
4	0.0	0.02	0.14	0.28	0.46	SF
5	0.0	0.04	0.15	0.28	0.49	SF
6	0.0	0.0	0.08	0.18	0.40	SF
7	0.0	0.03	0.20	0.40	0.56	SF
8	0.0	0.02	0.15	0.35	0.60	SF
1,3-bis(tripropylammonium)propane dibromide						
1	0.0	0.10	0.29	0.57	0.72	SF
2	0.0	0.0	0.13	0.41	0.65	SF
3	0.0	0.12	0.29	0.54	0.70	SF
4	0.0	0.06	0.13	0.41	0.63	SF
5	0.0	0.04	0.13	0.38	0.63	SF
6	0.0	0.03	0.07	0.22	0.56	SF
7	0.0	0.12	0.29	0.49	0.72	SF
8	0.0	0.06	0.20	0.43	0.74	SF

On control plates solvent compositions of 0 to 60% methanol gave steaks from origin to solvent front. With 80% methanol an improvement in spot shape and chromatography was seen whilst at 100% methanol all compounds migrated at the solvent front.
* For key see experimental section
SF=Solvent front

TLC on Silica Gel

As was observed for paraffin coated silica gel, any attempt to perform chromatography on silica gel in the absence of ion-pair reagents resulted in the test compounds chromatographing at, or near, the solvent front. Coating the plates with either the bistrimethyl or bistriethyl reagents gave a slight reduction in R_F when 100% water was used as mobile phase, but nowhere near as great a reduction as obtained on the paraffin coated plates described above. Between 20 and 80% methanol in the solvent gave high, and fairly uniform R_F values for both reagents. However, the use of 100% methanol as solvent produced a large reduction in R_F for all of the test compounds. This result is similar to that observed with paraffin coated

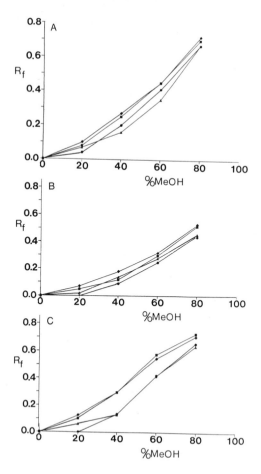

Fig. 2. IP–RP–TLC on paraffin coated silica gel of 2,4–dihydroxybenzoic acid (■), 2,6–dihydroxybenzoic acid (●), gentisic acid (◇) and salicylic acid (▲). Methanol-water solvent systems were used with plated impregnated with either 1,3-bistrimethyl (A); 1,3-bistriethyl (B), or 1,3-bistripropylammonium (C) ion-pair reagents.

plates. In contrast the bistripropyl reagent showed no significant reduction in R_F for any solvent composition, whilst spot shape was grossly distorted.

Chromatography using dichloromethane-methanol mixtures on ion-pair coated silica gel also revealed major differences in the properties of the bistriethyl and bistrimethyl reagents on the one hand and the bistripropyl on the other. Thus the bistriethyl and bistrimethyl ion-pair reagents were similar and gave good chromatography over the range 0 to 100% methanol in the mobile phase. The results obtained for both of these compounds were similar to those observed in our earlier studies[4] on the bistrimethyl reagent. The bistripropyl reagent gave results little different to the control silica gel and was only usable with 40% or less of methanol in the mobile phase.

Table 2. Variation of R_F with Solvent Composition of 8 Organic Acids for Paraffin coated Silica Gel on IP-TLC with 1,3-bistrimethyl; 1,3-bistriethyl and 1,3-bistripropylammonium IP-Reagents

% Methanol	0	20	40	60	80	100
Compound*			R_F			
1,3-bis(trimethylammonium propane dibromide						
1	0.44	0.56	0.66	0.74	0.58	0.23
2	0.17	0.38	0.53	0.75	0.71	0.44
3	0.41	0.53	0.66	0.64	0.58	0.26
4	0.27	0.45	0.53	0.69	0.47	0.31
5	0.36	0.49	0.52	0.59	0.49	0.31
6	0.18	0.33	0.42	0.54	0.49	0.24
7	0.35	0.51	0.53	0.61	0.47	0.18
8	0.12	0.42	0.52	0.58	0.46	0.09
1,3-bis(triethylammonium)propane dibromide						
1	0.26	0.44	0.63	0.69	0.52	0.33
2	0.06	0.22	0.54	0.62	0.64	0.63
3	0.30	0.44	0.64	0.68	0.60	0.41
4	0.15	0.30	0.50	0.61	0.61	0.44
5	0.30	0.38	0.54	0.60	0.50	0.38
6	0.80	0.22	0.40	0.56	0.5	0.37
7	0.27	0.42	0.60	0.65	0.49	0.36
1,3-bis(tripropylammonium)propane dibromide						
1	0.31	0.57	0.69	-	-	-
2	0.06	0.25	0.59	0.66	0.8	0.56
3	0.28	0.53	0.69	-	-	-
4	0.16	0.37	0.62	-	-	-
5	0.36	0.51	0.67	-	-	-
6	0.12	0.25	0.56	-	-	-
7	0.33	0.56	0.66	-	-	-
8	0.12	0.42	0.66	-	-	-

On control plates (no IP-reagent) all compounds ran at the solvent front.
- Spot shape so poor that R_F values could not be determined.
* For key see experimental section.

DISCUSSION

The properties of the bistriethyl and bistrimethyl bolaform ion-pair reagents are unique, and quite unlike those of any of the other ion-pair reagents which we have studied. The reduction in R_F seen with water-methanol mobile phases on silica gel and paraffin coated silica gel, and the ability to use these compounds for "normal-phase" separations on silica gel with dichloromethane-methanol mixtures are not properties of conventional ion-pair reagents such as tetra-n-butylammonium or cetrimide. However, as the length of the alkyl chain attached to the quaternary nitrogen is increased from methyl and ethyl to propyl the unusual "bolaform" behavior is lost and the bistripropyl reagent behaves on the whole as a normal ion-pair reagent.

The working hypothesis which we have used to rationalize the behavior of the bistrimethyl and bistriethyl compounds assumes that one of the quaternary nitrogens interacts strongly with a silanol on the surface of the silica gel, fixing the reagent in place, whilst the remaining quaternary nitrogen is left to interact with the charged acidic group on the test compounds. If this model is accurate then differences in behavior between the bistripropyl reagent and the other two compounds may partly reflect increased steric hindrance of the positively charged nitrogen in the former, which reduces its ability to interact with acidic silanols compared to the bistrimethyl and bistriethyl reagents. This model describes what occurs on silica gel and on paraffin coated silica gel. On C_{18} bonded silica gel all three bolaform reagents exhibit relatively "normal" behavior, with no evidence of the reduction in R_F and "normal phase" chromatography seen with high concentrations of methanol in the mobile phase. This difference may, in part, be due to the reduced number of silanols available following C_{18} bonding and perhaps also to restricted access to the residual silanols. The latter results both from steric effects, and also from the difficulty of a highly charged polar reagent penetrating the lipophilic C_{18} phase. In this respect it is perhaps note-worthy that the best spot shapes on C_{18} bonded plates were obtained for the bistripropyl reagent which, as we have speculated above, may be due to the charged nitrogens being better shielded by the bulkier side chain in this reagent compared to the others.

REFERENCES

1. S. Lewis and I. D. Wilson, J.Chromatogr., 31:133 (1984).
2. I. D. Wilson, J.Chromatogr., 354:99 (1986).
3. J. A. Troke and I. D. Wilson, J. Chromatogr., 360:236 (1986).
4. R. J. Ruane, I. D. Wilson, and J. A. Troke, J.Chromatogr. 368:168 (1986).

A NOTE ON: A PRELIMINARY INVESTIGATION OF THE INFLUENCE OF

THE STATIONARY PHASE IN ION-PAIR THIN-LAYER CHROMATOGRAPHY

R. J. Ruane and I. D. Wilson

Department of Safety of Medicines
ICI Pharmaceuticals Division
Mereside, Alderley Park, Macclesfield
Cheshire, SK10 4TG, UK

INTRODUCTION

Ion-pair (IP) reagents are routinely used for the chromatography of polar ionisable compounds in high performance liquid chromatography (HPLC). However, the application of these compounds to the separation of polar substances by thin-layer chromatography (TLC) has received much less attention (see refs 1 to 5 for some applications). In previous studies[4-8] we examined the use of quaternary ammonium IP-reagents as an aid to the TLC of some polar organic acids on a limited range of stationary phases (silica gel, C_{18} bonded silica gel and paraffin coated silica gel). Here we describe the results of preliminary studies undertaken using some of the other commercially available stationary phases with a range of ion-pair reagents. The phases investigated were C_2, C_8, aminopropyl (NH_2), cyanopropyl (CN) and diphenyl bonded silica gels, all of which were compared to a C_{18} bonded material for the chromatography of four aromatic acids as described below.

EXPERIMENTAL

E. Merck C_2, C_8, aminopropyl and cyanopropyl bonded glass backed high performance (HP)-TLC plates (10 x 10cm) were purchased from BDH Ltd (Poole, UK). Merck C_{18} bonded TLC plates (glass backed 20 x 10cm) were also obtained from BDH Ltd. Whatman diphenyl bonded TLC plates (glass backed, 20 x 20cm) were a gift from the manufacturer (Whatman Ltd, Maidstone, UK). All plates incorporated a fluorescent indicator and substances were visualized using a UV lamp at 254nm. Before use the plates were cut to size (5 x 10cm) using a diamond tipped glass cutter and then either dipped in a 0.1 M solution of the appropriate IP-reagent in methanol or used without further pretreatment.

Test acids were applied to the plates using 1 μl glass capillaries as a solution ($\sim$1mg ml^{-1}) in methanol. Ascending chromatography was performed in glass tanks 10 x 10 x 5cm. Solvent systems consisted of either methanol-water 1:1 for control and IP-coated plates or 0.1M IP-reagent in methanol-water 1:1 for untreated plates.

Tetra-n-butylammonium bromide, tetramethylammonium chloride and cetyl-trimethylammonium bromide (cetrimide) were obtained from Fisons Ltd (Loughborough, UK) whilst 1,3-bis(trimethylammonium)propane dibromide was synthesized as described previously[6].

The test acids used in these experiments were 2,6-dihydroxybenzoic acid, benzoic acid, p-chlorobenzoic acid and hydroxyhippuric acid. These compounds were purchased from Aldrich (Gillingham, UK), the Sigma Chemical Co. Ltd. (Poole, UK) or BDH Ltd. (Poole, UK).

RESULTS AND DISCUSSION

The test compounds were chromatographed with the ion-pair reagent either coated onto the plate (by dipping in a methanolic solution of 0.1 M reagent) or present in the solvent (0.1 M). The resulting R_F values were then compared with those obtained in control experiments where the test compounds were chromatographed in the absence of reagent. These results are summarized below.

In the absence of any ion-pair reagent all four of the test compounds ran at or near the solvent front on the aminopropyl, cyano and diphenyl modified silicas. On the C_2, C_8 and C_{18} bonded phases the compounds did not run at the solvent front and a general trend towards lower R_F with increasing alkyl chain length was observed (Figure 1). It should be noted that, certainly in the case of the C_{18} bonded plates, this solvent composition (methanol-water 1:1) is one of the few which could be used successfully for the chromatography of the test compounds. Either increasing the methanol content above 60% or decreasing it to below 40% often caused the compounds to run as badly distorted, elongated, streaks. Whether this is also the case for the C_2 and C_8 plates has yet to be determined.

The inclusion of ion-pair reagents in the system, either on the plate or in solution in the mobile phase, had with one exception (see below), no effect on the results obtained with aminopropyl bonded plates. On the cyanopropyl bonded plates significant reductions in R_F were often observed, but spot shape was usually poor, with large diffuse spots generally obtained. The largest effects observed were with cetrimide coated onto C_2, C_8, C_{18} and diphenyl bonded plates (Figure 2). Lesser effects were seen when cetrimide was present in solution and this is probably explicable in terms of the likely retardation of the reagent, which is somewhat lipophilic, relative to the solvent front. This would result in relatively low concentrations of ion-pair reagent being available at the point of contact between the sample and the advancing mobile phase to ion-pair with the test compounds. In contrast, for tetramethylammonium bromide, dipping the plates was slightly less effective than including the reagent in the solvent for C_8 and C_{18} bonded plates and much less effective on diphenyl and cyanopropyl plates (Figure 3). In contrast to cetrimide this reagent is a very polar water soluble compound which is unlikely to be much retained by the stationary phase. Thus on dipped plates it is probable that this ion-pair reagent would rapidly be eluted up the plate by the advancing solvent front, leading to a rapid depletion of the amount of reagent available for ion-pairing with the test compounds. The presence of tetramethylammonium bromide in the solvent however, would seem to ensure that sufficient ion-pair reagent was always available, and significant reductions in R_F values were obtained compared to both the control and dipped plates. Interestingly, when this reagent was coated onto C_2 bonded plates the migration of the solvent up the plate was almost completely inhibited. This is contrary to our usual experience where the presence of an ion-pair reagent on the plate appears to increase the rate of solvent migration (presumably by acting as a detergent). For the bolaform reagent 1,3-bis-

172

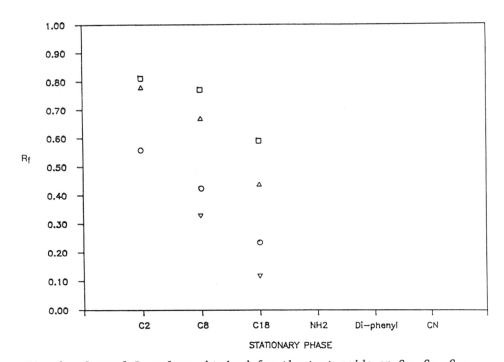

Fig. 1.   Control R_F values obtained for the test acids on C_2, C_8, C_{18}
aminopropyl (NH_2) cyanopropyl (CN) and diphenyl bonded plates in
the absence of ion-pair reagents. Key: 2,6 dihydroxybenzoic acid
□, benzoic acid ○, p-chlorobenzoic acid ▽, hydroxyhippuric acid
△ :-
The same symbols are used in subsequent figures, however, in
Figures 2-5 a solid symbol (i.e. ●) indicates the presence of
IP-reagent in the solvent whilst an open symbol (i.e. ○) indicates
that the reagent is present coated onto the plate.

(trimethylammonium)propane dibromide very similar results were obtained on
C_8 and C_{18} bonded plates whether the reagent was in the solvent or coated
onto the plated.   Once again no migration of the solvent was observed for
C_2 plates coated with the reagent.   Interestingly this reagent is the only
one for which any effect on the aminopropyl bonded plates was observed and
a significant reduction in R_F values was obtained compared to the control
(Figure 4).   For tetra-n-butylammonium bromide best results are once again
obtained for plates which had been coated with the reagent (Figure 5)
probably reflecting the greater lipophilicity of this compound compared to
tetramethylammonium bromide.

As well as the general effects described above it should be noted that
the relative migration order of the test compounds was often observed to
depend on whether the reagents were coated onto the plate or present in the
solvent.   Whilst we have, as yet, performed insufficient experiments to
enable us to forward a plausible explanation for these effects such phenomena are clearly of use if changes in the selectivity of a system are required.

CONCLUSION

In this preliminary study we have briefly examined whether IP-TLC with
quaternary ammonium reagents can be performed on a variety of stationary

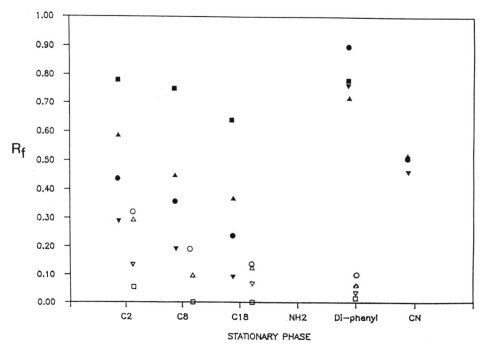

Fig. 2. The effect of using cetrimide as an ion-pair reagent on the R_F values of the test acids.

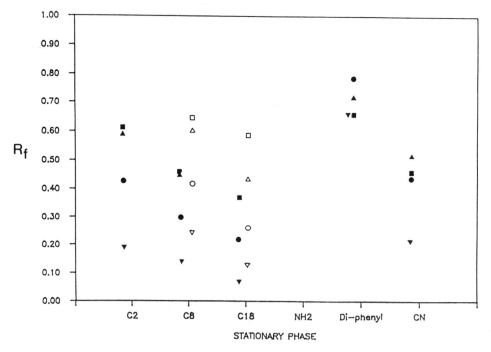

Fig. 3. The effect of using tetramethylammonium bromide as an ion-pair reagent on the R_F values of the test acids.

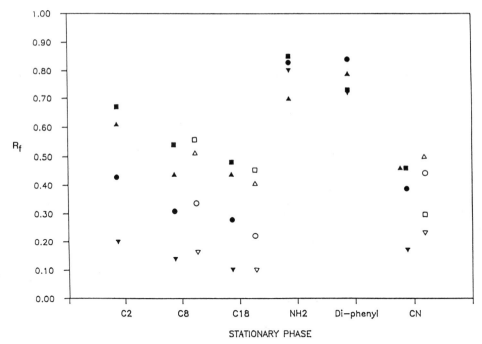

Fig. 4.   The effect of using 1,3-bis(trimethylammonium)propane dibromide as an ion-pair reagent on the R_F values of the test acids.

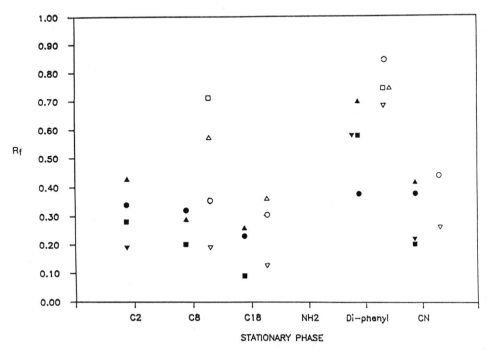

Fig. 5.   The effect of using tetra-n-butylammonmium bromide as an ion-pair reagent on the R_F values of the test acids.

phases. Clearly, with the exception of the aminopropyl bonded plates, such chromatography is possible. However, the situation is complex with the best results for a particular stationary phase depending upon the type of ion-pair reagent used, and whether it is coated onto the plate or present in the solvent.

Further studies are now in progress to define the importance of various factors for IP-TLC on these stationary phases.

REFERENCES

1.   G. Szepesi, Z. Vegh, Sz. Gynlay and M. Gazdag, J.Chromatog., 290:127 (1984).
2.   W. Jost and H. E. Hauck, J.Chromatogr., 264:91 (1983).
3.   H. M. Ruijten, P. H. Van Amsterdam and H. de Bree, J.Chromatogr., 252:193 (1982).
4.   S. Lewis and I. D. Wilson, J.Chromatogr., 312:133 (1984).
5.   I. D. Wilson, J.Chromatogr., 354:99 (1986).
6.   J. A. Troke and I. D. Wilson, J.Chromatogr., 360:236 (1986).
7.   R. J. Ruane, I. D. Wilson and J. A. Troke, J. Chromatogr., 368:168 (1986).
8.   R. J. Ruane and I. D. Wilson, This volume.

APPLICATIONS

A SENSITIVE HIGH PERFORMANCE THIN-LAYER CHROMATOGRAPHY

METHOD FOR THE DETERMINATION OF GR 38032F, A WEAKLY

FLUORESCENT COMPOUND, IN PLASMA

P.V. Colthup

Department of Biochemical Pharmacology
Glaxo Group Research Limited
Ware, Herts, UK

SUMMARY

GR 38032F is a novel, selective and potent 5-hydroxytryptamine$_3$ (5HT$_3$) receptor antagonist which is being developed currently for the treatment of certain psychiatric and gastrointestinal disorders. A sensitive high-performance thin-layer chromatographic (HPTLC) method for the determination of GR 38032F, a weakly fluorescent compound, in plasma is described. The endogenous background from plasma is minimized by way of a selective solid phase extraction procedure and a further clean-up on the HPTLC plate. The sensitivity is maximized by applying the entire extract from a 1ml plasma sample to the plate in a carefully selected solvent. The method is accurate and precise down to 1ng/ml in plasma. It has been used to analyze plasma samples from a bioavailability study in man.

INTRODUCTION

The drug GR38032F (Figure 1), 1, 2, 3, 9-tetrahydro-9-methyl-3[2-methyl-1H-imidazol-1-yl)methyl]-4H-carbazol-4-one hydrochloride, is a novel, selective and potent 5-hydroxytryptamine$_3$ (5-HT$_3$) receptor antagonist which is being developed currently for the treatment of certain psychiatric and gastrointestinal disorders (1). Before the pharmacokinetics of GR 38032F could be investigated a method for the determination of the compound in plasma was required. It was anticipated that the required sensitivity would be 1ng/ml.

The physical and chemical properties of GR 38032F were considered before deciding which chromatographic technique to use for its determination. GR 38032F has an ultraviolet absorption maximum at 310nm in 0.1M HCl, and in solution has a weak native fluorescence (λEx = 322nm, λEm = 420nm in 0.1M HCl). The fluorescence of GR 38032F in solution was not strong enough to give sufficient sensitivity for the development of a high-performance liquid chromatographic (HPLC) method with fluorescence detection. HPLC with ultraviolet absorbance detection was considered. GR 38032F could not be derivatised to improve its detection by UV absorbance or fluorescence after HPLC, or to make it suitable for analysis by gas-liquid chromatography (GLC).

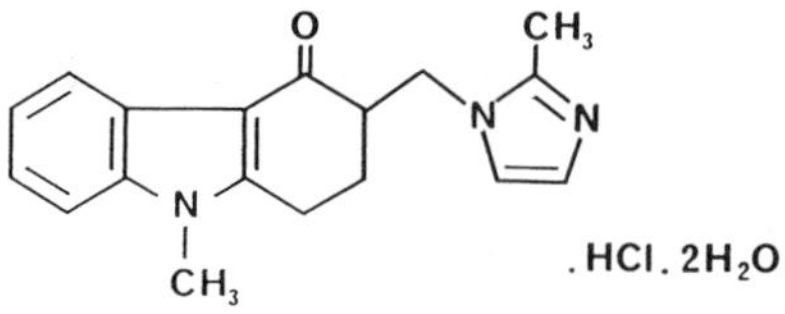

Fig. 1. GR 38032F, 1, 2, 3, 9-tetrahydro-9-methyl-3[(2-methyl-1H-imidazol-1-yl)methyl]-4H-carbazol-4-one hydrochloride

When GR 38032F was dry on a silica gel thin-layer chromatography plate the fluorescence was more intense and 0.5ng could be detected by fluorescence densitometry. It was considered that detection by fluorescence would give greater selectivity than ultraviolet absorbance detection, therefore high-performance thin-layer chromatography (HPTLC) was selected for the development of an assay for GR 38032F in plasma. In order to achieve the required sensitivity it was necessary to apply the whole extract from a 1ml plasma sample to the HPTLC plate.

This paper reports a technique in which the entire extract obtained after solid phase extraction of a 1ml plasma sample was applied to an HPTLC plate. Application of the technique to the determination of GR38032F in plasma is described. The method is precise and accurate down to 1ng/ml in plasma and has been used to analyze plasma samples from a study to determine the bioavailability of GR 38032F in man.

EXPERIMENTAL

Chemicals, Standards and Materials

GR 38032F was supplied by the Pharmaceutical Sciences Division of Glaxo Group Research. Methanol and acetonitrile, both HPLC grade, were from Rathburn Chemicals (Walkerburn, UK); methanol, ethyl acetate and 35% ammonia solution (Aristar ®) and hydrochloric acid, sp.gr. 1.18 (AnalaR®) were from BDH (Poole, UK); chloroform (Pronalys AR®) was from May and Baker Limited (Dagenham, UK).

Merck glass backed silica gel 60 HPTLC plates (10 x 20cm) without fluorescent indicator were from BDH; Bond Elut® CN sample preparation cartridges (100mg) were from Jones Chromatography (Llandradach, UK).

Selection of a Solvent for Sample Application

The sensitivity of the method to determine GR 38032F in plasma relies on the application of a large volume of an extract to the HPTLC plate without the loss of sensitivity and resolution which might occur if the resultant spot was large. This was achieved by selecting a solvent for spotting in which the analyte had an Rf of approximately zero.

A suitable solvent was selected after following the procedure described as follows. GR 38032F was dissolved in small amounts of a number of solvents. A spot (3 x 2μl) of each sample was applied by Microcap® (2μl, Drummond, Scientific Supplies, London, UK) to a Merck silica gel 60 HPTLC plate with fluorescent indicator that had been pre-developed with methanol. The plate was then inspected under an ultra-violet lamp and the spot diameters were measured. From this experiment acetonitrile was selected as the most suitable solvent in which to apply GR 38032F to the HPTLC plate.

Sample Preparation

Samples were prepared for analysis by use of solid phase extraction. A vacuum box was used to draw samples and solvents through the extraction cartridges. Bond Elut CN sample preparation cartridges (100mg) were washed sequentially with 1ml methanol and then twice with 1ml of distilled water. The cartridges were not allowed to dry. After the second wash with water sufficient vacuum was applied to remove the excess water from the cartridges. Hydrochloric acid (0.5N, 50μl) was applied to the cartridge immediately before a plasma sample (1ml). The sample and acid were drawn through the cartridge together, the eluate was discarded and the cartridge allowed to dry. The cartridge was then washed sequentially with water (2 x 1ml) and acetonitrile (2 x 1ml), then allowed to dry. GR38032 base was eluted with 1% ammonia in chloroform (v/v) (2 x 1ml) into a 2ml Eppendorf centrifuge tube (Sarstedt, Leicester, UK) and the solvent removed at 45°C on a Savant Speed Vac concentrator (Stratech Scientific Limited, london, UK).

Sample Application

Prior to the application of samples, the surface of the HPTLC plate was cleaned by pre-developing the plate with methanol. Samples were applied 0.5cm from the bottom edge of the plate (Merck silica gel 60 without fluorescent indicator, 10 x 20cm) and 0.55cm apart. The entire extract from a 1ml plasma sample was applied to the plate. The technique is summarized in Figure 2.

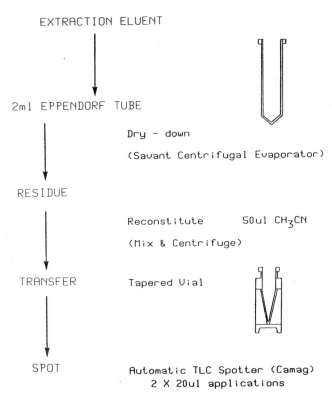

Fig. 2.   Summary of the procedure used to apply the entire extract from a 1 ml plasma sample to the HPTLC plate.

The dried extract in the Eppendorf centrifuge tube was reconstituted in 50µl acetonitrile, centrifuged (Eppendorf 5412 centrifuge, 1.0min), and transferred to a tapered vial using a P200 Gilson pipette (Anachem, Luton, UK). Quantitative transfer of the extract was achieved by this technique. The extract was applied to the HPTLC plate using an automatic TLC sample applicator (Camag, Muttenz, Switzerland). One application of 20µl was made and the spotting sequence was repeated to apply a second 20µl on the initial spot. Application of 40µl from a sample of 50µl using the automatic spotter meant that in practice almost all of the sample was applied. Small losses occurred in the pre-dose and excess volumes taken up by the spotter, also some evaporation of the extract solvent took place between the first and second applications of sample. Sample application was carried out in the dark because GR 38032 base was found to be light sensitive when applied to silica gel.

Chromatography

Chromatography was carried out in a horizontal linear development chamber (Camag). The HPTLC plates were first developed with acetonitrile for 4.5cm beyond the origin to remove co-extracted material which otherwise interfered with the subsequent chromatography of GR 38032 base. The plates were then redeveloped with ethyl acetate - methanol - distilled water (6 : 4: 1 by vol.) to 3.5cm beyond the origin, and dried for 1h at room temperature in the dark before being scanned.

Detection and Quantification

Plates were scanned from origin to solvent front with a Camag TLC Scanner II using fluorescence detection, a monochromator wavelength of 313nm (Mercury lamp), a K400 cut off filter, micro-optics and a scan speed of 0.5mm/sec. The signal output was recorded on a Trivector Trilab 2000 chromatography data system.

Standard solutions of GR 38032F in plasma over the range 1 to 10ng base/ml and a control plasma sample were analyzed, peak heights were recorded, and calibration lines constructed using quadratic least squares regression. GR 38032 base concentrations in quality control samples (spiked plasma samples) and in unknown samples were quantified by comparison with these standard lines. Samples containing GR 38032 base at concentrations greater than 10ng/ml were analyzed after dilution with control plasma.

RESULTS AND DISCUSSION

Sample Application

The smallest spot sizes were obtained when GR 38032F was applied to the HPTLC plate in acetonitrile or ethyl acetate (Table 1). Acetonitrile was selected in preference to ethyl acetate because it dissolved the dried residue from the extraction more easily. Acetonitrile could also be used to pre-develop the HPTLC plate after sample application. This removed co-extracted endogenous material to the solvent front without causing migration of the analyte.

Quantification

Typical chromatograms which were obtained from the analysis of GR 38032F in plasma are shown in Figure 3. Comparison of the chromatograms from the 1ng/ml standard and the plasma blank shows that GR 38032 can be distinguished clearly from endogenous material at 1ng base/ml in plasma.

Table 1. Spot Sizes obtained by Spotting
         GR38032F from different Solvents

Solvent	Spot Diameter (mm)
Methanol	6.0
Acetonitrile	2.0
Acetone	3.0
Isopropyl Alcohol	3.5
Ethyl Acetate	2.0
Chloroform	5.0
Dichloromethane	3.0

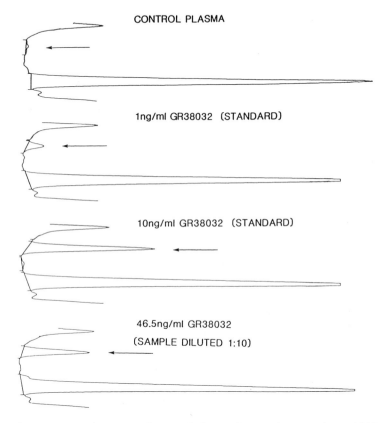

Fig. 3. Chromatogram traces obtained from the analysis of GR 38032
        calibration standards in plasma and a human plasma sample.
        (Human plasma sample taken 2 hours after 16 mg oral dose).

Precision and Accuracy

     Intra and inter-assay precision and accuracy were determined by
analysing spiked plasma samples. The intra-assay precision and accuracy
were determined on two separate occasions (days 1 and 2, Table 2). The
results showed that the precision was good; coefficients of variation being
less than 10%. The bias results were less than 10%, which indicated that
the method had acceptable accuracy. The inter-assay precision and accuracy
data (Table 3) were obtained from 24 independent assay runs carried out by
two analysts working independently. The results showed that good accuracy

Table 2. Intra-Assay Precision and Accuracy of the HPTLC Assay for
         GR 38032 in Plasma

Day	Nominal Concentration (ng/ml)	n	Observed Concentration (mean ± SD) (ng/ml)	Coefficient of Variation (%)	Bias (%)
1	1.5	5	1.38 ± 0.13	9.4	-8.0
1	4.7	5	4.42 ± 0.27	6.1	-6.0
1	9.4	5	8.64 ± 0.63	7.3	-8.1
2	1.0	5	1.09 ± 0.07	6.5	+9.0
2	4.7	5	4.78 ± 0.07	1.4	+1.7
2	9.4	5	9.22 ± 0.84	9.1	+1.9

Table 3. Inter-Assay Precision and Accuracy of the HPTLC Assay for
         GR 38032 in Plasma

Nominal Concentration (ng/ml)	n	Observed Concentration (Mean ± SD) (ng/ml)	Coefficient of Variation (%)	Bias (%)
2.0	48	1.94 ± 0.27	14.1	3.0
5.0	48	4.79 ± 0.53	11.0	4.2
8.5	48	8.26 ± 0.66	8.0	2.8

was achieved, bias results all being less than 5%. The precision was not
as good as that obtained from a single assay run but was less than 15% at
2ng/ml which is near the limit of quantification of the assay. It was
found that with a high and reproducible extraction efficiency (mean 93.9%,
standard deviation 0.6%, n=6, at 10ng/ml) and quantitative transfer of the
reconstituted extract to the HPTLC plate, the use of an internal standard
did not improve the precision of the method.

Analysis of Human Samples

    Analyses were carried out as part of a study in healthy volunteers to
determine the bioavailability of GR 38032F in man. Plasma samples were
taken at various times after oral dosing by solution (16mg) and an intravenous dose (8mg). The results obtained from one subject are shown in
Figure 4. These results underlined the importance of maximizing the sensitivity of this assay. Validation of the method down to 1ng/ml in plasma
enabled the pharmacokinetics to be followed to 26 hours after an oral dose
and 24 hours after an intravenous dose.

CONCLUSIONS

    A sensitive assay in plasma with good accuracy and precision has been
developed for GR 38032F, a compound which itself has only a weak native
fluorescence. The sensitivity was achieved by minimizing the endogenous
background from the sample matrix and maximizing the proportion of the
sample which was analyzed. This method demonstrates the potential for
increasing the sensitivity of other existing HPTLC assays where at present
only a small percentage of the sample is applied to the plate for analysis.

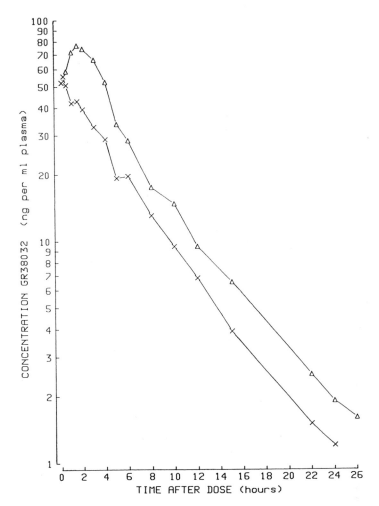

Fig. 4. Plasma concentrations of GR 38032 base from a volunteer given an
intravenous and oral dose. X intravenous (8 mg), △ oral solution
(16 mg).

ACKNOWLEDGEMENTS

The author would like to thank Mr. C. C. Felgate, Department of Biochemical Pharmacology, Glaxo Group Research for his assistance in the
analyses reported in this paper.

REFERENCES

1. R. T. Brittain, A. Butler, I. H. Coates, D. H. Fortune, R. Hagan, J.
M. Hill, D. C. Humber, P. P. A. Humphrey, S. J. Ireland, D. Jack,
C. C. Jordan, A. Oxford, D. W. Straughan and M. B. Tyers,
Br.J.Pharmac., 90, 87P (1987).

185

THIN-LAYER CHROMATOGRAPHY-DENSITOMETRY AS A POWERFUL METHOD

FOR THE STANDARDIZATION OF MEDICINAL PLANT EXTRACTS

M. Vanhaelen* and R. Vanhaelen-Fastré

ULB, Institut de Pharmacie
Laboratoire de Pharmacognosie, B205-4
Bd Triomphe, 1050 Bruxelles, Belguim

SUMMARY

TLC-densitometry is proposed as an alternative method to HPLC and GLC for the standardization of crude medicinal plant extracts. Results obtained from a number of medicinal plants studied in the laboratory show that, in most cases, TLC-densitometry is a more convenient method than HPLC and GLC. The pre-purification steps essential to the application of HPLC and GLC are considerably simplified or can be avoided. Moreover, the chromatograms obtained during quantitative analysis are useful, both for extract characterization as an overall fingerprint, and for the detection of the possible adulteration or degradation of the drugs.

INTRODUCTION

Since the plant kingdom represents an almost inexhaustible source of biologically active compounds, some of our most useful drugs are derived from plants; in addition, many of their constituents have been used as models for the hemi-synthesis or the synthesis for many other therapeutic agents. We can hope that the intense interest in the field of herbal medicine now shown by the general public will ultimately influence the pharmaceutical industry to renew its interest in the study of plants whose useful properties have still to be discovered.

As a result of modern purification and pharmacological screening methods, most medicinal plants used in the past have found their way into current medicine as purified substances rather than in the form of older galenical preparations of crude extracts. However, an increased interest in these latter extracts is now being observed.

The wide variety of organic substances that are elaborated and accumulated by plants requires highly sophisticated methods for their separation, purification, identification and quantitative determination.

It is the purpose of this study to show the value of the thin layer chromatography-densitometry method for the quantitative determination of biologically active constitutents in several medicinal plants.

Three types of difficulty can be expected for such determinations. Firstly, the biologically active constituents of plants are not always clearly defined or are generally considered to be a complex mixture of several plant constituents. Secondly, the active constituents of plants are mixed with other ballast compounds which generally create interference in determinations. Thirdly, as the substances determined are of natural origin, a high variability of content is usual, thus, the methods proposed must be sufficiently versatile and specific to take such large variations into account.

Under these circumstances, the use of chromatographic methods are obviously essential, and gas liquid chromatography (GLC) and high performance liquid chromatography (HPLC) both appear to be potent candidates for these quantitative determinations. The results provided by both methods are usually very accurate, and the coefficients of variation are generally lower than 1%. However, they do require tedious pre-purification steps which, in most cases, can lead to a loss of the constituents to be determined. Therefore, though it is less accurate, quantitative TLC, which usually requires less sample preparation, provides a useful alternative to GLC and HPLC methods. For example, in a recent study, Prosek has shown that the determination of thebaine in two hundred samples of Papaver bracteatum required ten hours using TLC-densitometry, and about one hundred using HPLC[1].

Another feature of TLC-densitometry is the use of chromatograms as overall fingerprints of crude extracts and not, as in HPLC or GLC, as parts of these extracts analyzed in the elution conditions selected by the operator. Therefore, the probability of detecting possible degradation or adulteration of the drug is higher by TLC.

In addition, many post-chromatographic reagents may be exploited to provide compound-specific or class-specific colors or fluorescences in order to enhance specificity and/or sensitivity. UV-VIS spectrometry (either fast scanning or diode array) which has only recently introduced into HPLC detection methods can be applied "in situ" to check the purity of the separated compounds on TLC, and to determine the optimum wavelength for scanning. Of course, the sensitivity of detection in TLC is lower than in HPLC, but the applied volumes to be analyzed using both methods are quite different: one μl and less in TLC-densitometry, compared with 10 to 25μl in HPLC. Generally, constituents which are present in plant extracts at a concentration not lower than 1% can be quantified without difficulty, when the constituents are fluorescent, this value could be as low as 0.05%. Factors involved in the precision of the TLC-densitometry method have been well documented in a number of books and publications dealing with this subject[2-7].

Most TLC-scanners are now capable of measuring absorbance, reflectance, fluorescence and fluorescence quenching, and provide the spectra of individual spots "in situ". The precision of densitometric measurements is high; however, twenty-five repetitive measurements of a well-resolved spot in the fluorescence mode indicate that the coefficient of variation of these measurements can rise by 1%, this value is obviously higher when the chromatograms are complex.

The sample application step is of critical importance for reproducible results. Devices are now available which can automatically apply volumes of 50 nanoliters and more with a precision of 1%. Contact spotting or spraying are both of interest. The spraying technique is especially useful for the application of bands. The coefficients of variation observed with the measurements of such bands may be twice as high in comparison with the measurements of spots. However, in the case of very complex mixtures, this mode of sample application greatly improves the resolution and accuracy of quantification by eliminating the interference of "ballast" constituents or other constituents of interest, in addition, the distribution of the compound within the band is more uniform and remains uniform during development. I would like to point out two aspects of the sample application which are considered less frequently. The first one concerns the distance between the initial spot or band and the surface of the mobile phase. This parameter involves the reproducibility of the position of the sample from the lower edge of the plate and the level of the mobile phase in the tank. The second factor involves the nature of the solvent used for the sample application. In the best conditions, it should not favor the migration of the constituents around the spot or the band during application, and must be at least less polar than the mobile phase in order to obtain a pre-concentration effect of the constituents in the solid phase and a distribution within this phase which is as small as possible. Such an effect can be illustrated by the chromatography of quinine: the coefficient of variation in the densitometric measurements of this alkaloid is greater when the polarity of the solvent used for the application increases.

Since its discovery, TLC has evolved into an important analytical tool with the development of a range of alkyl-bonded phases and of small sized adsorbent particles. Improvements in resolution, sensitivity and reproductibility are the main characteristics of HPTLC. However, in some experiments, we have observed that the reproductibility of the densitometric measurements was higher when conventional plates were used. It is also interesting to note that measurements carried out in the migration direction provide lower coefficients of variations than perpendicular measurements.

In addition to the traditional development conditions, involving a single development with the mobile phase, a number of new techniques have been developed such as circular and anti-circular methods, programmed multiple development, continuous development and overpressurized TLC. Considering the reasons for the popularity of TLC, namely its simplicity, speed and modest demand on equipment, all our procedures involve conventional development alone, without tank saturation.

RESULTS AND DISCUSSIONS

As is shown in Table 1, a number of applications of the TLC-densitometric method have been carried out in our laboratory, and these include several classes of biologically active compounds such as alkaloids, iridoids, saponins and phenols.

The first application which will be described is the determination of sennosides A and B in Cassia spp[8]. Recent studies on the laxative activity and metabolism of the anthracenic derivatives of Cassia have unequivocally confirmed that the most active constituents of these drugs are sennosides A and B. The aim of our study was the selection of optimum culture conditions for African Cassia spp to enhance the high production of anthracenic compounds. Numerous plant samples cultivated in different ecophysiological conditions were determined and compared by TLC-densitometry. Earlier conditions used for the chromatographic separation of sennosides and chosen for the Senna monograph of European Pharmacopeia were improved using silica gel buffered at pH 7.5 to suppress the distortion of the spots.

On the other hand, the previously described detection conditions provide very poor sensitivity, useless for densitometric measurements.

Table 1. Biologically Active Constituents from Plant Material Determined by TLC-densitometry

Class of biologically active constituents	Plant Material	Determined Constituent(s)
Alkaloids	Rauwolfia vomitoria	Reserpine, rescinnamine, ajmaline
	Cinchona spp.	Quinine
	Datura spp.	Hyscyamine, hyoscine
	Hyoscyamus spp.	Hyoscyamine, hyoscine
	Holarrhena floribunda	Conessine
	Cola nitida	Caffeine
Iridoids	Gentiana lutea	Gentiopicrin
	Olea europea	Oleuropein
	Picrorrhiza kurroa	Picrosides I and II
Saponins	Glycyrrhiza glabra	Glycyrrhizin
	Aesculus hippocastaneum	Aescin
	Acanthopanax senticosus	Eleutheroside E
	Panax spp.	Ginsenosides
Phenols	Equisetum arvense	isoquercitrin
	Cynara scolymus	Cynarin
	Hammelis virginiana	Gallic acid, tanins
	Salix alba	Salicin
	Fraxinus excelsior	Fraxin
	Silybum marianum	Sylibin
	Arctostaphylos uva-ursi	Arbutin
	Betula alba	Hyperosid
	Uncaria gambir	Catechin
	Crataegus oxyacantha	Vitexin-2"-O-rhamnosid procyanidins
Anthracenics	Hypericum perforatum	Hypericin, pseudohypericin
	Cassia spp.	Sennosides A and B
Miscellaneous	Stevia rebaudiana	Stevioside
	Piper methysticum	Kawain

Thus, a highly sensitive method for the detection of the dianthrone derivatives is proposed. It involves their "in situ" reduction by spraying an aqueous solution of sodium borohydride in the presence of sodium stannite. This reduction produces yellow-green fluorescent spots which are too unstable for further chemical investigation. The sodium stannite strongly inhibits their oxidation and thus allows reproducible measurements of the fluorescent spots. The densitometric data are compared with those obtained by HPLC and show little differences in the results and the coefficients of variation. Our second example within this group is Hypericum perforatum[9]. The crude extract of this plant contains hypericin and pseudohypericin. These compounds are responsible not only for the sedative properties of the plant but also for its photosensitive effects, they are present in very low concentrations of about 0.05%. Fortunately, these compounds exhibit a very sensitive red fluorescence when they are excited at 313nm. They were extracted from the crude extract using pyridine, and their separation was performed on a reversed-phase TLC adsorbent with acetonitrile as solvent, the separations were obtained over a distance of 50mm in less than 5 min.

With regard to iridoids, Gentiana lutea represents an important plant for the pharmaceutical and food industries. Bitter constituents are mainly localized in the roots of the plant, they stimulate gastric secretion and improve the appetite. Gentiopicrin is considered to be sufficiently characteristic, other more bitter and possibly more important iridoids such as amarogentin, amaroswerin and amaropanin were not measurable by the proposed method without preliminary fractionation. The separation of the constituents was achieved on silica gel using 1,2-dichloroethane-methanol-water (39:10:1 v/v), with detection at 280 nm[9].

Oleuropein, a hypotensive constituent from the leaves of Olea europea, can be separated and determined under similar conditions using UV detection at 245nm[9].

Aescin corresponds to a complex mixture of saponins related to the barringtogenol nucleus esterified by low molecular organic acids and by an osidic chain constituted of glucuronic acid and glucose units. It is used successfully in the prevention and treatment of various peripheral vascular disorders. It is present in the seeds of Aesculus hippocastaneum in very high concentrations. Atypically, the constituents of aescin were not separated intentionally so as to allow a comparison of the densitometric results with the commercially available standard[9]. The versatility of the TLC-densitometric method is clearly demonstrated here. The GLC method is not applicable and HPLC would only be applicable with difficulty because of the absence of chromophores available for UV detection. The use of a chromogenic reagent must be carefully studied, only low concentrations of the spraying reagent have to be used, especially when aggressive compounds like sulphuric acid are chosen. The best solvent for spraying, in our experience, is methanol, it allows a very good dispersion of the reagents and thanks to a low boiling point, enables large volumes of solutions to be sprayed onto the plate. In comparison with other reagents, the spraying of an extemporaneous mixture 1:1 of a 1% vanillin methanolic solution and a 5% sulphuric acid methanolic solution followed by heating at 120° provides a very good detection method for aescin and other saponins. Generally, it should be emphasized that the use of chromogenic reagents increases the coefficients of variation of the densitometric measurements and must be avoided as far as possible. This effect could be attributed to a possible non-homogenous spraying of the reagents, and a similar reaction of the compounds to be detected.

Other applications in this class of biologically active constituents include two plants which are now attracting public attention, namely, Panax spp (Ginseng) and Acanthopanax senticosus (syn. Eleutherococcus senticosus). They have been claimed to enhance a non-specific resistance of the organism and the recuperative power of the body and act as both a stimulant and a sedative. The wide variety of commercial preparations of Ginseng include the powdered root, capsules and tablets prepared from the powdered root or its extracts and teas, cigarettes, chewing gum and sweets. Culture conditions, species used and the treatment of the roots after collection induce important modifications in the content of their active constituents which in their turn, are related to a very complex mixture of a number of saponin glycosides termed ginsenosides. The main ones are based on the aglycons oleanolic acid, (20s)-protopanaxadiol and (20s)-protopanaxatriol; glucose, rhamnose, arabinose and xylose are present in varying amounts in the osidic chain. The main saponins Rb_1, Rb_2, Rc, Re, Rd and Rg_1 are separated under the conditions described in Figure 1[10].

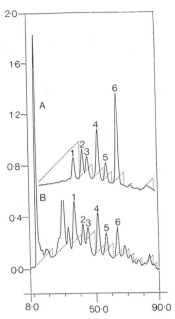

Fig. 1. Scanning profile of a spray-dried extract of Panax ginseng (B) compared with that of a synthetic mixture of ginsenosides (A). Adsorbent: silica gel 60F$_{254}$ HPTLC plate. Mobile phase: 1,2-dichloroethane-ethanol-methanol-water (65:22:22:7 v/v). Detection: the chromatogram was sprayed with a mixture 1:1 of a 1% vanillin methanolic solution and a 5% sulphuric acid methanolic solution, heated at 120°C for 5 min and measured at 530 nm after color stabilization (10 min). 1: ginsenoside Rb$_1$, 2: ginsenoside R$_2$, 3: ginsenoside Rc, 4: ginsenoside Re, 5: ginsenoside Rd, 6: ginsenoside Rg$_1$.

The heterosidic compounds from Acanthopanax senticosus are quite different. One of them is a glycosidic saponin derived from oleanolic acid but the main active constituent is eleutheroside E, a glycosidic lignoid formed by syringaresinol linked to two glucose units. The separation of this eleutheroside is achieved under the same experimental conditions as those selected for the Ginseng extracts[10]. However, in this case, UV detection is not specific because the concentration of eleutheroside E is very low in the crude extract and there is a lot of interference in the chromatograms. The use of a vanillin-sulphuric acid reagent must be considered only as a compromise between specificity and sensitivity for eleutheroside E detection. From the comparison between HPLC and TLC-densitometry, it appears that the results obtained by the two methods are very similar except that TLC-densitometry gives a coefficient of variation which is twice as high, and an apparent sensitivity ten times lower. However, the number of determinations per hour using the HPLC method is considerably lower than with the TLC-densitometry method because frequent washings of the HPLC column are essential to recover its initial performance.

Phenolic compounds are widely distributed in plants. Antihepatotoxic constituents are found to be present in the seeds of the milk thistle, Sylibum marianum; they are related to flavanolignans and, some years ago, put an end to the sceptical assertion that there is no effective drug therapy for liver diseases. Four flavanolignans have been isolated, mainly silybin, isosilybin, silydianin and silychristin, and the mixture of these four is termed silymarin. Silybin has been shown to be more active than the other three constituents and was thus selected for determination[9].

Another well-known antihepatotoxic drug is the horticultural artichoke, Cynara scolymus, in this plant, the most active constituent is a depside cynarin, together with a number of caffeic acid derivatives. It is very easy to separate and to determine this constituent from other compounds, which appear on hydrolysis of cynarin as chlorogenic acid or caffeic acids (Figure 2).

Extracts prepared from the dried flowers, fruits and leaves of Crataegus oxyacantha are used in minor forms of heart disease, heart failure and cardiac arythmia. These therapeutical properties are related to flavonoids and oligomeric procyanidins. The main flavonoid, vitexine-2"-O-rhamnoside, was selected for determination. Separation was obtained using the mobile phase of ethyl acetate, formic acid, acetic acid and water (50:4.5:4.5:11 v/v) (Figure 3). After determination, the spraying of a 1% diphenylborinate solution allowed the visualization of vitexin-2"-O-rhamnoside and other flavonoids of interest, such as hyperin. Other conditions allow the determination of hyperin, the main flavonoid of Betula alba leaves (Figure 4) or the determination of isoquercitrin in Equisetum arvense (Figure 5). The determination of oligomeric procyanidins from Crataegus oxyacantha is more critical especially because standards are not commercially available and/or unstable. It was decided to compare the chromatograms of the extracts with a standard of catechin which, with the vanillin-hydrochlorhydric acid reagent, gives a specific red color; oligomeric procyanidins give the same reaction. A complex mixture of solvents including propanol, 1-butanol-acetonitrile, dichloroethane, formic acid and water is selected to obtain a reasonable separation of these polymers (Figure 6).

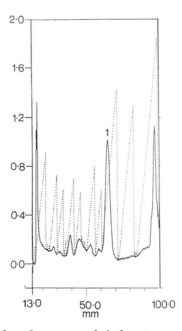

Fig. 2. Scanning profile of a spray-dried extract of Cynara scolymus. Adsorbent: silica gel 60F$_{254}$. Mobile phase: ethyl acetate-formic acid-actic acid-water (50:4.5:4.4:11v/v). Detection: UV at 325 nm. 1. Cynarin.

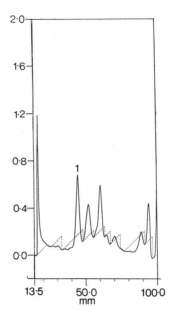

Fig. 3.   Scanning profile of a spray-dried extract of <u>Crataegus oxyacantha</u>.
Adsorbent: silica gel 60F$_{254}$ HPTLC plate. Mobile phase: ethyl
acetate-formic acid-acetic acid-water (50:4.5:4.5:11v/v).
Detection: UV at 335nm. 1. Vitexin-2"-O-rhamnoside.

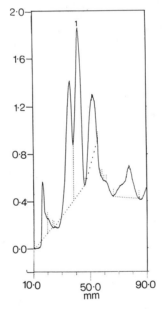

Fig. 4.   Scanning profile of a spray-dried extract of <u>Betula alba</u> leaves.
Adsorbent: Cellulose F$_{254}$ for HPTLC. Mobile phase: acetic
acid-water (15:85v/v). Detection: UV at 370nm. 1: Hyperin.

The last application in this section will be the determination of
fraxin in <u>Fraxinus excelsior</u> leaves. This coumarin glycoside might be
involved in the antirheumatic properties of the drug to the extent that the
analgesic and anti-inflammatory properties of 6,7-dimethylesculetin iso-

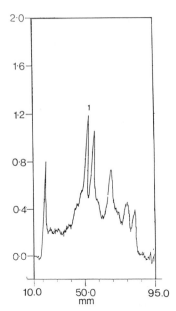

Fig. 5. Scanning profile of a Equisetum arvense spray-dried extract.
Adsorbent: RP-18 F_{254}s. Mobile phase: acetonitrile-water-acetic
acid (30:70:1 v/v). Detection: UV at 360 nm. 1. Isoquercitrin.

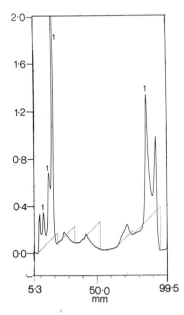

Fig. 6. Scanning profile of a spray-dried extract of Crataegus oxyacantha.
Adsorbent: silica gel $60F_{254}$ HPTLC plate. Mobile phase:
1-propanol-1-butanol-acetonitrile-dichloromethane-water-formic
acid (15:15:15:12.5:10:2 v/v). Detection: Vis at 510 nm after
spraying a 1% vanillin solution in hydrochlorhydric acid. 1:
procyanidins.

lated from <u>Artemisia capillaries</u> has been demonstrated "<u>in vivo</u>". Our first method involved the use of silica gel as adsorbent and spot measurement[9] by fluorometry, however, we established that the fluorescence emitted by fraxin in these experimental conditions was not stable enough for quantitative work. The use of a reversed-phase RP-18 stationary phase, a mobile phase consisting of a mixture of water and acetonitrile and a diluted potassium hydroxide ethanolic solution as reagent eliminated this problem (Figure 7). It is generally observed that the stability of the fluorescence is better when reversed-phases such as RP-18 or RP-8 are used. It is likely that the lipophilic phase linked to the silica gel prevents the degradation of the fluorescent compounds and quenching by oxygen; it must be emphasized that the 1μg of any compound enclosed in 4mm² of the thin-layer is actually dispersed on 1m² of the adsorbent, and is thus in a very favorable condition to undergo photo-chemical or chemical degradation.

Our first example concerning alkaloids is the determination of three alkaloids from <u>Rauwolfia vomitoria</u>[11]. A number of alkaloids have been isolated from Rauwolfia root-barks. Reserpine and rescinnamine are ester alkaloids related to the principal medicinal use of this drug, i.e. the treatment of hypertension and mental disorders, ajmaline is a non-esterified alkaloid and is widely used as an anti-arythmic drug and also as a precursor of semi-synthetic drugs. From previous studies on the TLC of Rauwolfia alkaloids, and because of the large basicity and polarity differences between ajmaline and reserpine-rescinnamine, it is evident that TLC cannot be used any more than HPLC to determine all the alkaloids with a one-step chromatographic development. The mobile phase used for reserpine-rescinnamine also induces a low ajmaline migration, in these chromatographic conditions, "<u>in situ</u>" UV spectrometry of the ajmaline spots in the extracts indicates that this alkaloid is apparently well resolved, but further investigations lead to the conclusion that other alkaloids with similar Rf values and UV spectra interfere. This explains the need for

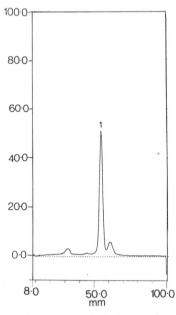

Fig. 7. Scanning profile of a spray-dried extract of <u>Fraxinus excelsior</u>. Adsorbent: silica gel RP-18 $F_{254}s$. Mobile phase: acetonitrile-water (3:7v/v). Detection: fluorometry, excitation at 365 nm after spraying a 1% KOH methanolic solution. 1. Fraxin.

another chromatographic procedure such as HPLC, which allows a comparison of the assay results. We also observed an extensive degradation of reserpine and rescinnamine on silica gel, so that the addition of α-tocopherol acid succinate to standard solutions was found essential in order to perform the accurate determination of these two alkaloids. Most of the previously described TLC assays for reserpine and rescinnamine were probably distorted because degradation was not taken into account. Because of its easier reproductibility, the fluorescence of the reserpine and rescinnamine spots is best developed by keeping the plates in the dark for 15 hours. This treatment probably yields stable 3-dehydroderivatives. Again, the results obtained by HPLC and TLC-densitometry (the fluorescence mode for reserpine and rescinnamine, UV absorption for ajmaline) are very similar. The analysis of many samples of Rauwalfia cultivated in different culture conditions was easily achieved by TLC-densitometry. For the purpose of the same type of comparison, a great number of samples of Holarrhena floribunda were analyzed for their content of conessine, a steroidal alkaloid which shows very interesting amoebicidal properties but also severe adverse effects. In spite of this toxicity, the use of Holarrhena in traditional African medicine is still observed. Thus the standardization of the drug is considered to be imperative. The HPLC method was totally inapplicable for this alkaloid, and only GLC may be used for comparison with the TLC-densitometric results. Conessine is easily separated from other minor steroidal alkaloids. As no chromophore is present in the conessine structure the Dragendorff reagent was used together with the iodoplatinate reagent, which improves the sensitivity of coloration up to tenfold and discolors the yellow background of the chromatograms[12]. This method was also successfully applied to the determination of conessine in callus cultures of Holarrhena floribunda[13]. TLC-densitometry of the main alkaloids found in mydriatic Solanaceae species, as previously published, have resulted in poor sensitivity or the high instability of the colors produced by means of the detection reagents described. The aim of the work is again the study of the ecophysiological factors which influence the production of hyoscyamine and hyoscyne in the leaves, fruits and seeds of Datura spp[14]. The procedure was also successfully applied to the determination of the same alkaloids in hairy root cultures of Hyocyamus and Datura strains. Transformed root cultures, the so-called hairy roots, are obtained following the insertion of T-DNA from the root inducing (Ri) plasmid of Agrobacterium rhizogenes into the plant genone. They have the two advantages of fast growth and organ differentiation. The production of alkaloids is affected by the biochemical variability between strains initiated from different plantelets, between strains issuing from the same plant, and by the composition of the culture medium. The analytical method involves a simple extraction step of the alkaloids, avoiding liquid-liquid partitions. Hyoscyamine and hyoscyne were extracted in a centrifuge tube using diethylether after alkalification with calcium hydroxide. The ether extract was then applied to a column filled with diatomaceous sulphuric acid supporting earth. The nonalkaloidal materials were removed by elution, firstly with diethylether, and then with chloroform, and the alkaloids were then eluted with ammonia-saturated chloroform. The search for a sensitive method to detect the alkaloids was essential. We therefore proposed a modified Van Urk's reagent used previously by Karawya et al.,[15] for "in vitro" colorimetric determinations of hyocyamine and hyoscyne, with the solvents being adapted to obtain a homogeneous spraying of the TLC plates. The heating temperature of 100°C was found to be optimal for color development without charring the alkaloids. The reddish derivatives contrasted well on a colorless background and were found to present an absorption maximum at 495 nm; the concentration of 0.2 to 2μg of alkaloid base/ml spotted gives a linear calibration graph, with a limit of detection of ca 50 nanograms.

The determination of caffeine in <u>Cola nitida</u> extracts requires no purification and is very easy to perform with the experimental conditions described in Figure 8. Again the use of UV spectrometry to check "in situ" the purity of the spots and the comparison of the results with HPLC determinations are essential.

The last application to be described is the determination of quinine, the major alkaloid found in <u>Cinchona spp</u>. barks. This method was recently developed in our laboratory in order to have a convenient procedure for the analysis of a large number of samples per day. The extraction step was simplified as far as possible as follows: after alkalification with sodium hydroxide, the powder was refluxed with toluene for three hours. This time was sufficient to take all the alkaloids into solution. This solution was diluted, and then applied directly to the plates. The mobile phase selected affords the efficient separation of the quinine from other alkaloids. After development, the plates were sprayed with a diluted methanolic solution of sulphuric acid to enhance the fluorescence of the quinine and measurements were carried out perpendicularly to the direction of mobile phase migration (Figure 9). The results calculated in these conditions were identical to those obtained with HPLC, but with a lower coefficient of variation. The good results yielded by this method can be attributed to four factors:

(1)   The use of toluene as a solvent provides a favorable pre-concentration of the alkaloid on the adsorbent.

(2)   The mobile phase efficiently separates the quinine and leads to low Rf values and the reduced diffusion of the spot during development.

(3)   The solutions of the alkaloidal extracts are very diluted: therefore, no distortion of spot size can be observed in comparison with standards.

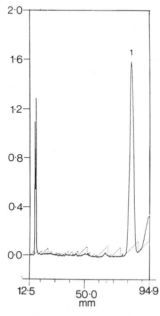

Fig. 8.   Scanning profile of a spray-dried extract of <u>Cola nitida</u>. Adsorbent: silica gel 60 F_{254}. Mobile phase: ethyl acetate-methanol-17% ammonia (80:17.5:7.5 v/v). Detection: UV at 273 nm. 1: Caffeine.

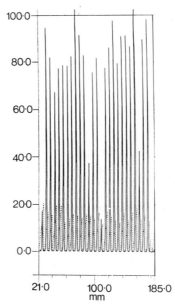

Fig. 9. Scanning profile (measurements are perpendicular to the migration
direction) of a chromatogram used for the determination of quinine
in <u>Cinchona</u> bark extracts. Adsorbent: silica gel 60. Mobile
phase: toluene-diethylether-diethylamine (55:35:10 v/v).
Detection: fluorometry, excitation at 365 nm after spraying a 5%
sulphuric acid methanolic solution. Standard concentrations: 0.25
(lower limit) to 2 mg (upper limit)/10 ml toluene. Spotted
volumes: 1 μl. <u>r</u> values of the calibration graphs: > 0.999.
Coefficient of variation (10 determinations): < 3%.

(4)   The small size of the spots and their good alignment on the
      plate allow the measurement of a large number of spots on the
      same plate.

CONCLUSION

      All these applications show clearly that, when correctly applied and
controlled by other chromatographic methods, TLC-densitometry is very
versatile and convenient for the analysis and the quality control of plant
extracts, for the selection of optimal culture conditions, for the selection of industrial plants and for the analysis of secondary metabolites in
plant cell or organ cultures. Its use for the routine determination of
synthetic drugs must be re-evaluated as a result of the development of
modern instruments capable of automatic spot application and rapid
densitometric measurements.

ACKNOWLEDGEMENTS

We thank Mr. B. Carlier for his skilful technical assistance.

REFERENCES

1. M. Prosek, M. Katic, and M. Pukl, <u>in</u>: "Quantitative Thin-Layer
    Chromatography And Its Industrial Applications," Laszlo R. Treiber

ed., Chromatographic Science Series, vol. 36, Dekker, New York, p. 275 (1987).

2. E. J. Shellard "Quantitative Paper And Thin-Layer Chromatography," Academic Press, London, (1968).

3. J. C. Touchstone, "Quantitative Thin-Layer Chromatography," Wiley, New York, (1974).

4. J. C. Touchstone and J. Sherma, "Densitometry In Thin-Layer Chromatography, Practice And Applications," Wiley, New York, (1979).

5. J. C. Touchstone and D. Rogers, "Thin-Layer Chromatography, Quantitative Environmental and Clinical Applications," Wiley, New York, 1980.

6. R. E. Kaiser, "Proceedings Of The Second International Symposium On Instrumental HPTLC," Institute for Chromatography, Bad Dürkheim, Federal Republic of Germany, (1982).

7. Laszlo R. Treiber, "Quantitative Thin-Layer Chromatography And Its Industrial Applications, Chromatographic Science Series, vol. 36, Dekker, New York, (1987).

8. P. Duez, M. Vanhaelen, R. Vanhaelen-Fastré, M. Hanocq and L. Molle, J.Chromatogr. 303:391 (1984).

9. M. Vanhaelen and R. Vanhaelen-Fastré, J.Chromatogr. 281:263 (1983).

10. M. Vanhaelen and R. Vanhaelen-Fastré, J.Chromatogr. 312:497 (1984).

11. P. Duez, S. Chamart, M. Vanhaelen, R. Vanhaelen-Fastré, M. Hanocq and L. Molle, J.Chromatogr. 356:334 (1986).

12. P. Duez, S. Chamart, M. Vanhaelen, R. Vanhaelen-Fastré, M. Hanocq and L. Molle. J.Chromatogr. 351:140 (1986).

13. L. Bouillard, J. Homès and M. Vanhaelen, Phytochem. in press.

14. P. Duez, S. Chamart, M. Hanocq, L. Molle, M. Vanhaelen and R. Vanhaelen-Fastré, J.Chromatogr. 329:415 (1985).

15. M. S. Karawya, S. M. Abdel-Wahab, M. S. Hifnawy and M. G. Ghourab, J.Ass.Offic.Anal.Chem. 58:884 (1975).

A NOTE ON: TRIGLYCERIDE ANALYSIS USING SILVER NITRATE AND 2-PHASE

2-DIMENSIONAL THIN-LAYER CHROMATOGRAPHY

A. S. Ritchie and M. H. Jee

Cadbury Schweppes plc
Reading, UK

INTRODUCTION

The analysis of Triglycerides using not only thin-layer chromatography with flame ionisation detection (TLC-FID) using the Iatroscan technique, but also the use of silver nitrate multi-phase TLC for the separation of triglyceride isomers is briefly described.

Triglycerides, the major constituent of most fats and oils, consist of a triol, glycerol, in which the three hydroxyl groups are esterified with a fatty acid. It is important to note that the three hydroxyl groups are not equivalent. From the point of view of the physical chemistry of the fats, the positional isomerism, which results from esterification of the primary and secondary hydroxyl groups with different fatty acids, is more important than the optical isomerism, which results from the two carbon atom being chiral when the 1- and 3- alcohols are esterfied differently. The result of esterification of the three positions with different permutations of fatty acids is that triglycerides can vary in both carbon number (total number of carbon atoms in the fatty acid portions of the glycerides) and also in the ratios and positions of the fatty acids. Conventional analysis using GC or HPLC gives an analysis either by carbon number, by total fatty acid, or by equivalent carbon number. This information is limited in what it tells the analyst about the nature of the fat. As Table 1 shows, animal fats, for example lard, can look similar to vegetable fats such as cocoa butter, using these analytical techniques. However, as shown in Figure 1 the major triglycerides of cocoa butter and lard are very different, in that the position of the unsaturated fatty acid (oleic) is in the 2-position in cocoa butter but in the 1 (3)- position in lard.

HPLC methods do not readily lend themselves to modification of the stationary phase. Silver nitrate, the most obvious modifying agent, shortens column life drastically. Both the silver nitrate and the column are very expensive. Two workers at Unilever, Dallas and Padley[1], succeeded in separating triglyceride isomers differing only in the relative positions of the unsaturated fatty acids, using silver nitrate - TLC (argentation chromatography). The mechanism of silver nitrate - TLC is that the silver ions complex with double bonds in the triglycerides, which has the effect of retarding migration of compounds proportionately to the number of double bonds. The position of the double bonds in the glycerides also has an effect on this retardation. A specific method using a mixture

Table 1. Analytical Data

	Lard	Cocoa Butter
Triglycerides		
C50	26	22
C52	56	46
C54	22	30
Fatty Acids		
Palmitate	30	28
Oleate	41	35
Stearate	16	34

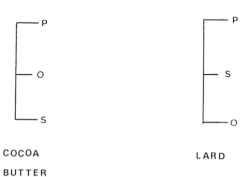

COCOA
BUTTER

LARD

Fig. 1. Major triglycerides of cocoa butter and lard.
Key: P, palmitic; O, oleic; S, stearic.

of chloroform and toluene as a solvent is necessary to separate mono-unsaturated isomers differing only in the position of the oleic acid; in fact the technique is such that it only works on certain brands of TLC plate.

The main difficulty with TLC is that it is not easy to quantify components after separation. The alternatives available are: visual standard comparison, densitometry, and scraping/extraction followed by GC analysis. The Iatroscan (developed by Iatron Laboratories in Japan) provides an alternative approach to this problem by carrying out the thin-layer chromatography on cylindrical TLC rods instead of plates. After development the rods are passed through a flame ionisation detector, which pyrolyses the sample in the flame and detects the ions formed in the same way as a GC-FID.

RESULTS AND DISCUSSION

Many workers have separated fatty acids or triglycerides using Chromarods impregnated with silver nitrate. We, however, have succeeded in separating the positional isomers of mono-unsaturated triglycerides described earlier using a solvent mixture of chloroform-benzene-diethyl ether (70:30:1.5). Thus, Figures 2 and 3 show the type of separations that can be obtained. The "Chromarods", unlike HPLC columns or TLC plates so used, are reusable. They can be washed with nitric acid and then re-impregnated with silver nitrate several times with no loss of resolution. However, washing leaves some silver ions on the rods so they cannot subsequently be reused except for silver nitrate TLC. The advantages of the Iatroscan for analyses of this type are:

1. Time. 10 analyses take approximately 2 hours of which about 1 hour is operator time.
2. Quantification. This is quite simple as the Iatrocan can be linked to a computing integrator.

There are however, some disadvantages. Accuracy is not as good as TLC when coupled with a densitometer. Using the Iatroscan minor components can be underestimated; for example a 25% mixture of the triglyceride PSO in POS (P, S and O as defined in Table 1) is reported by this method as 19%. Sensitivity is inferior to TLC/Densitrometry. Detection limit is 2 to 3% using the Iatroscan, whereas by TLC it is around 1%. It is up to the individual worker to weigh the pros and cons of the methods.

Multi-phase TLC has proved useful for the rapid profiling of Triglyceride mixtures using Whatman "Multi-K" TLC plates. The principle of multi-phase TLC is that components are separated in two different directions, as in conventional two-dimensional (2D) TLC, but it is separated in the different directions according to different parameters. One type of multi-phase plate, the Multi-K CS5 consists of a silica-gel plate with a strip, about 3cm wide of octadecyl bonded silica down one edge. Triglycerides can be separated firstly on the reversed-phase section of the plate according to the equivalent carbon number (ECN), defined below, by triple development in acetone/acetonitrile.

$$ECN = CN - 2DB$$

Where CN = carbon number

DB = number of double bonds

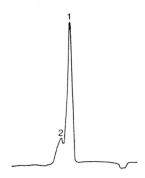

Fig. 2. Separation of symmetrical and unsymmetrical mono-unsaturated triglycerides using chloroform-benzene-diethyl ether (70:30:1.5 v/v). S, = saturated, U = monounsaturated. Key: 1, SUS; 2, SSU.

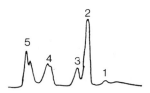

Fig. 3. Separation of cocoa butter/lard mixture using chloroform-benzene-diethyl ether (70:30:1.5 v/v). Key: 1, SSS; 2, SUS; 3, SSU; 4, Diunsaturates; 5, Triunsaturates.

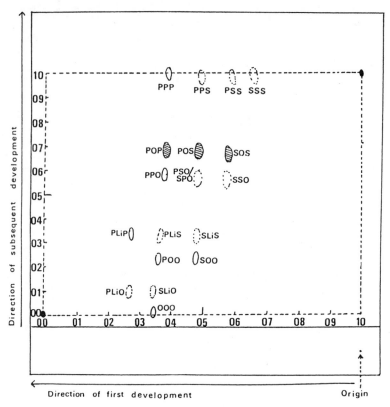

Fig. 4. Typical separation on a "Multi-K" TLC plate

The ratio of acetone and acetonitrile has to be varied according to the type of mixture being studied. For fats of the cocoa butter type a ratio of 80:20 has been found to be satisfactory. However, where fats containing large amounts of triglyceride of low ECN are analyzed, a higher proportion of acetonitrile is desirable. For example, a ratio of 60:40 is suitable for butter fat. Following development on the reversed-phase section, the TLC plate is impregnated with silver nitrate, and a second development at right angles to the first separates the glycerides according to the number and position of the double bonds. The result of this kind of separation is shown in Figure 4.

Identification of triglycerides is carried out using marker glycerides (trimyristolein, and triarachidin). Using the markers as corner points, a grid is constructed to calculate a reference point of each triglyceride. The main problem is that the location of the constituent triglycerides of the fat under analysis relative to the markers is variable; this is due to the multiple development techniques used, which tend to exaggerate small differences in R_f values. This problem can be solved by running simul- taneously samples of known composition on a separate TLC plate. As the solvent development times are identical this eliminates the variability in R_f values. HPLC provides similar information to this technique. However, using multi-phase TLC separation of the symmetrical and unsymmetrical monounsaturated triglycerides is again achieved, which is not readily achieved using HPLC.

CONCLUSIONS

Multiphase TLC gives a method for rapid profiling of triglycerides using relatively cheap raw materials and provides information not readily obtained by other methods. However, as with all TLC methods quantification of components is difficult, and indeed is particularly difficult using a two dimensional technique.

The two methods, argentation chromatography and multiphase 2D-TLC, described here can be seen to be complimentary to other chromatographic techniques. They are either more convenient or contain different information to that obtained using GC or HPLC.

REFERENCE

1. M. S. J. Dallas, and F. B. Padley, Lebensm. Wiss. Technol., 10:328 (1977).

A NOTE ON: SEPARATION AND QUANTIFICATION OF FUCHSIN BASIC USING REVERSED-PHASE HIGH PERFORMANCE THIN-LAYER CHROMATOGRAPHY

P. E. Wall

BDH Ltd
Broom Road
Poole BH12 4NN

INTRODUCTION

Thin-layer chromatography (TLC) has proved to be a useful technique for the separation of the components of basic fuchsin, new fuchsin and magenta crystalline. Commercial basic fuchsin has for some time been suspected, and is now known, to be a mixture of up to four methylated derivatives of a triaminotriphenylmethane base in varying concentrations[1] (see Figure 1). Previous papers have described TLC separation methods using silica gel 60, polyamide and reversed-phase silica gel layers for fuchsin analogs[2-4]. The purpose of this note is to present an improved method of separation with better resolution combined with less diffusion and to describe a reliable spectrodensitometric method of quantification for pararosanilin, one of the histologically important components of basic fuchsin.

In many staining procedures the results vary little with the composition of the dye. However, there are important methods where only pararosanilin gives stable, acceptable results, e.g.. the Feulgen & Schiff procedure for DNA[5] and preparation of aldehyde fuchsin for staining unoxidised pancreatic B Cells [6,7]. Both titanous chloride assay and UV analysis methods give results of total dye content, but they both assume only one component of known molecular weight is present[8]. Unfortunately most fuchsin basic labelled with the correct color index number for pararosanilin is a mixture of analogs. It is therefore possible that a total dye content of 98% for a specific batch has an actual pararosanilin content of less than 10%. For this reason there is a sound commercial reason to establish a reliable method of analysis for basic fuchsin and particularly pararosanilin.

MATERIALS AND METHODS

All reagents were provided by BDH Ltd, Poole, Dorset, England. Water and methanol were HiPerSolv grade. Formic acid was AnalaR grade and 1-pentanesulphonic acid sodium salt and industrial methylated spirit were reagent grade.

10 x 10cm pre-coated silica gel HPTLC RP8 glass plates were obtained from E Merck, Darmstadt, West Germany.

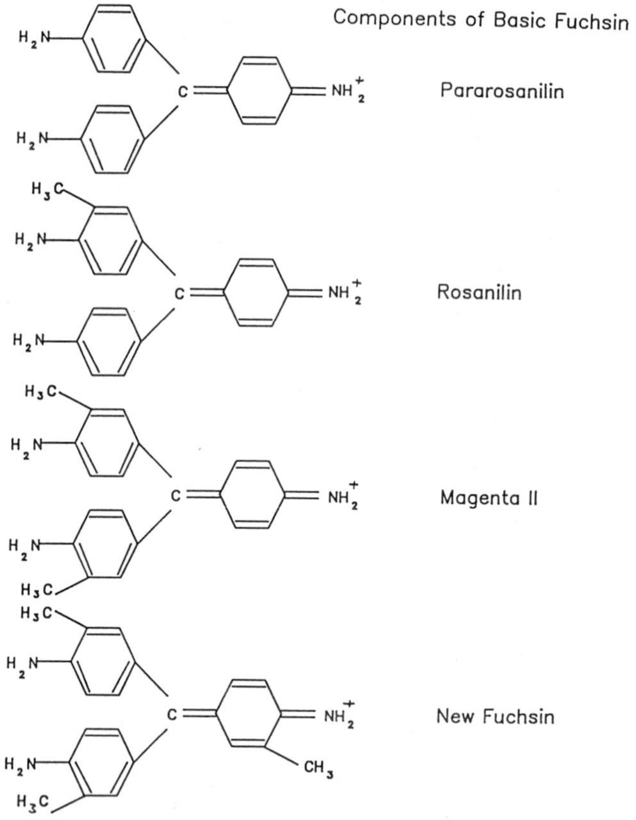

Fig. 1. Components of basic Fuchsin

Spotting of sample and reference solutions was achieved with a variable volume Nano-Applicator (50 to 230 nl) and a NANOMAT (Camag, Muttenz, Switzerland).

Glass N-chambers, saturated with solvent vapor, were used for chromatogram development. After development, the HPTLC plates were scanned with a spectrodensitometer (HPTLC/TLC Scanner I fitted with monochromator and mercury lamp, CAMAG, Muttenz, Switzerland).

Data interpretation and computation from the scanner was achieved with an HP 3390A integrator fitted with an I/O board and linked via an RS232 interface to an HP 86B computer with appropriate printer, plotter and I/O and plotter ROMS (Hewlett-Packard, Winnersh, Berkshire). A computer program was written in BASIC to manipulate data for calculation of Z_f, R_f, k, H, N and R_s (where Z_f is the migration distance of the solvent front, k is the velocity constant, H is the plate height, N is the number of theoretical plates and R_s is the resolution between peaks), to give a printed report of the results plus graphical presentation of peak height data, and calculation of percentage standard deviation.

Test samples and reference pararosanilin were prepared respectively for spotting by dissolving in a mixture of industrial methylated spirit and water (50:50 v/v) at a concentration of 0.1g/100ml. Complete solution was effected after a few minutes' shaking at room temperature. The reference standard solution was diluted respectively to 80%, 60%, 50%, 40% and 20%.

The test sample solutions and standards were applied to the silica gel
HPTLC RP8 layer using the Nano-Applicator and NANOMAT. Application was
made at 5 to 10mm intervals and the plate dried at 70°C for 3 to 5 minutes.

After extensive optimization work, the following solvent mixture was
found to give the best resolution, with the lowest rate of diffusion with
migration:- methanol-water-formic acid (75:20:5v/v). 1-Pentane sulphonic
acid sodium salt (2g/100ml) was added to the eluant to decrease peak
'tailing' effects. The eluant mixture was poured immediately after
preparation into the chromatography chamber lined with filter paper. The
chamber was then left to saturate and equilibrate with solvent vapor. The
HPTLC plates were developed vertically in the chamber, the solvent being
allowed to migrate to a distance of 80mm.

After development the sorbent layer was dried at 70°C (5 minutes).
The separated spots were scanned 'in situ' with the spectrodensitometer
using a slit width of 3mm, a mercury lamp source with the wavelength set at
540nm, and a scan speed of either 1 or 0.5mm/sec. For the reference
standard pararosanilin at different dilutions the computer plots the peak
height units against concentration. Statistically, the software finds that
an x-power curve gives the best 'fit' to the data obtained and on the basis
of this draws the appropriate plot and then calculates the test sample(s)
concentration (Table 1). The standard deviation of the method (n=7) was
0.51 (Table 2). Typical chromatograms are illustrated in Figure 2 for
samples from a variety of sources.

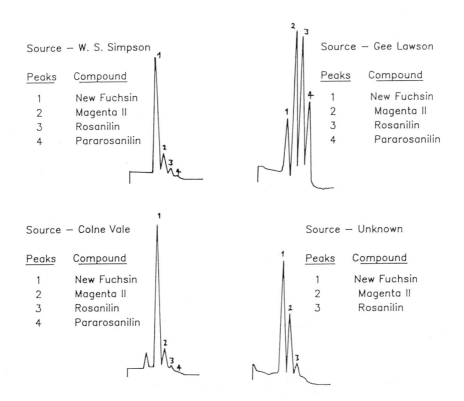

Fig. 2. Separation of commercial Fuchsin basics

Table 1. Pararosanilin Content For Samples

Test Sample	Peak Ht. Units	% Dye
1	446.4	19.4%
2	432.33	18.27%
3	452.63	19.88%
4	451.59	19.80%
5	710.63	44.03%
6	1080.1	92.14%

Table 2. Reproducibility and Standard Deviation of Pararosanilin

Run	Peak Ht. Units		
1	61658		
2	61849	MEAN	61531
3	60883		
4	61425	STANDARD DEVIATION =	315.43
5	61661		
6	61532	% STANDARD DEVIATION =	0.51
7	61709		

Measurements made by spotting volumes of 100nl being applied to the plate at 1cm intervals along one edge. The plate was then developed in the solvent mixture until the solvent front had migrated about 5cm. The spots were scanned at 540nm (mercury lamp) to obtain the peak height values.

DISCUSSION

Although 1-pentanesulphonic acid is normally used as an ion-pairing reagent, in the separation described it is more probably acting as a modifier on the silica surface. Apart from a slight retardation in migration of spots the main effect observed is a reduction in 'tailing' or 'streaking'. It is therefore suspected that, although the HPTLC layer is extensively silanised, such that only low concentrations of water can be accommodated (about 30%), excess silanol groups are interacting to some extent with the basic dye components. The ion-pair reagent prevents this occurring by interaction itself and/or causes layer formation.

The method gave reliable quantitative results for pararosanilin with a standard deviation of ± 1 to 2%. Good resolution of the other methylated 'impurities' and measurable R_F values were also obtained.

REFERENCES

1. K. Kovacs and J. B. Longley, J.S.C.Med.Assoc., 71:11 (1975).
2. T. Takeshita, N. Itoh, and Y. Sakagami, J.Chromatogr., 57:437 (1971).
3. G. S. Nettleton and A. W. Martin, Stain Technol., 54:213 (1979).
4. J. P. Koski, P. A. Heine and J. R. Pagel, J.Histotech., 2:119 (1979).
5. G. Clark, Staining Procedures, Williams and Wilkins, Baltimore/London, 4th ed., Ch.7, p. 201. (1981).
6. R. W. Mowry, Stain Technol., 53:141 (1978).
7. R. Ortman et al., J.Histochem.Cytochem., 14:104 (1966).
8. H. J. Conn, in: "Biological Stains," R. D. Lillie ed., ch.20, p. 582 (1977).

A NOTE ON: THIN-LAYER CHROMATOGRAPHIC PROCEDURES FOR THE

IDENTIFICATION OF PHARMACEUTICAL OILS AND FLAVORS

M. Postaire, J.J. Prat, P. Prognon
E. Postaire and D. Pradeau

Laboratoire de Contrôle de Qualité
Pharmacie Centrale des Hôpitaux
7, rue du Fer à Moulin, 75005 Paris, France

INTRODUCTION

Due to the frequent use of essential oils and flavors (both natural and artificial), in the manufacture and formulation of patent medicines, the correct identification of these substances is an important area for pharmaceutical quality control laboratories.

The literature contains relatively little information on this topic. Originally such substances were defined on the basis of their botanical origins, their methods of manufacture and their description. As early as 1880 Wallach[1] demonstrated, in a study of natural oils, that it was possible to characterize them by physico-chemical properties such as density and specific rotation etc.

Since that time, some analytical methods have evolved towards the use of modern techniques such as thin-layer chromatography (TLC)[2,3], gas liquid chromatography (GLC)[2,4], high performance liquid chromatography (HPLC)[5,6] and recently gas chromatography and mass spectrometry (GCMS) [7,8] which have been used in the study of the aromatic composition of essential oils.

For a quality control laboratory, it is important to have simple, quick, and easily applied methods directed towards the analysis of essential oils.

We propose a TLC system to enable profiles for pharmaceutical flavors to be obtained in this way and use this technique to identify the components found in medicines.

EXPERIMENTAL

Chromatography was performed on Kieselgel silica GF (E. Merck) TLC plates 2.5 x 10 cm with layers 0.25 mm thick.

Solvent systems were composed of mixtures of methanol, chloroform, sodium hydroxide (NaOH) and hydrochloric acid, (HCl). A total of 7 solvent systems were used as follows, 1, chloroform; 2, chloroform-methanol, 95:5;

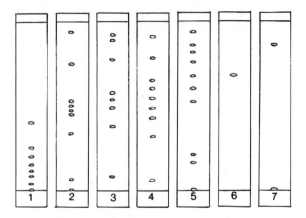

Fig. 1.   Chromatogram of a bitter orange oil.

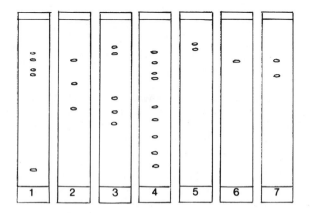

Fig. 2.   Chromatogram of a bergamot oil.

chloroform-methanol - HCl, 95:5; 3, chloroform-methanol - NaOH, 95:5;
chloroform-methanol, 90:10; 6, chloroform-methanol, 50:50; 7, methanol.
These solvent systems range in dielectric constant from 4.8 to 32.63 and in
eluotropic strength from 0.26 to 0.73.

Samples (1 and 5 µl) were spotted 0.5 cm from the lower edge of the
plate and developed for 9 cm. Plates were visualized under UV light at 254
nm.

RESULTS

Using the chromatographic systems described in the experimental section the identity and purity of the following raw materials have been
obtained:- lavender oil, lavendin oil, clove oil, eucalyptus oil, lemon
oil, citronnella oil, cinnamon oil, bergamot oil, peppermint oil, the
natural flavors of strawberry, rasberry, orange and bitter orange.

Identification and purity were established based upon the number of
spots and their respective R_F values in the various solvent systems used.
For example Figures 1 and 2 show chromatograms obtained from a bitter
orange oil (Figure 1) and a bergamot oil (Figure 2). For the bergamot oil
solvent system 4 gives the best separation with R_F values from 0.12 to

0.80. In this system 9 different constituents of the oil were detected
from the 119 found by GC-MS[8]. Comparison of the "fingerprint" obtained
for a sample with a standard can enable the detection of a possible fraud.
Comparison of Figures 1 and 2 show that there are large differences in the
fingerprint of the two oils and similar differences were seen for the other
oils examined. The detection of adulteration of natural flavors with
artificial flavors is thus possible as well as is the substitution of an
artificial oil for a natural one. The composition of the oils may not
necessarily be affected by the country of origin as, in the case of lemon
oils, no differences were seen with samples from either France or the USA.
However, when 3 different batches of citronnella oil were examined,
produced in 1983, 1984 and 1985, differences were noted in the presence of
certain high R_F spots.

Thin-layer chromatography has proved to be a very useful complementary
technique for use together with GLC and HPLC. The method has been found to
be both reproducible and inexpensive and should be included in the essential oils monographs of the relevant pharmacopoeia.

REFERENCES

1. Y. F. Pouchus, Thèse de 3 ème cycle. UER des Sciences Pharmaceutiques.
    Nantes, (1981).
2. A. DI. Giacomo, Labo.Pharma.Probl.Tech., 277:508 (1978).
3. H. H. Wisneski, J.Ass.Off.Agric.Chemist., 59:547 (1976).
4. Y. F. Pouchus, S. Drouet and M. Rouzet, Labo.Pharma.Probl.Tech. 30:319
    216 (1982).
5. C. N. Hensby, Clin.Exp.Derm., 3:355 (1978).
6. C. K. Shu, J. P. Walradt and W. I. Taylor, J.Chromatogr., 106:271
    (1975).
7. Y. Masada, Analysis of Essential Oils by Gas-Chromatography and Mass
    Spectra, Wiley, New York, (1976).
8. G. Mazza, J.Chromatogr., 362:87 (1986).

A NOTE ON: CHROMATOGRAPHIC STUDY OF SEVERAL AMINOGLYCOSIDE TYPE

ANTIBIOTICS BY OVERPRESSURE LAYER CHROMATOGRAPHY

K. Kovács-Hadady

Biogal Pharmaceutical Works
Debrecen
Hungary

INTRODUCTION

The chromatographic separation of the A, B and C components of neo-mycin in 2.5 M aqueous sodium chloride containing 30% of ethanol has recently been published.[1]. Cserháti et al.,[2] also published a thin-layer chromatographic (TLC) study of methylated amino acids using aqueous salt solutions as eluents.

By these earlier findings several questions are raised: e.g. what is the role of ethanol in the separation, what is the role of the salts and how do other aminoglycosides (tobramycin, apramycin, kanamycin A and B) behave? How can the overpressure layer chromatography (OPLC), developed by Tyihák et al.,[3-5], be used for the separation in case of aqueous salt solutions and what is the difference between the results of OPLC and TLC. This note describes the results of experiments designed to address some of these questions.

EXPERIMENTAL

The separations were carried out with high performance thin-layer chromatographic silica gel plates (Whatman Chemical Separation Inc. USA) For the OPLC three sides of the layers were impregnated with Impres UP polymer suspension from Labor MIM (Hungary).

TLC chambers were saturated with aqueous salt solutions for 16 hours, using filter papers.

OPLC was carried out with a Chrompres-10 overpressure layer chro-matograph (Labor MIM, Hungary) at 40°C, cushion pressure: 12 bars, eluent flow rate: 0.75 ml/min. Aqueous solutions of lithium chloride, sodium chloride, potassium chloride, ammonium chloride, magnesium chloride, cal-cium chloride, potassium bromide and potassium iodide were applied as eluents.

Antibiotics studied: neomycin A (as the hydrochloride), neomycin B and C, tobramycin, apramycin, kanamycin B as bases (BIOGAL working standards), kanamycin A as sulphate (USP reference standard). Aqueous sample solutions

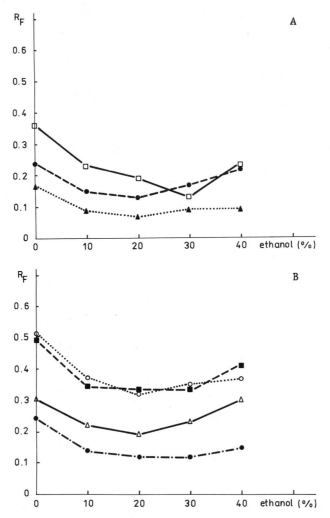

Fig. 1. Effect of ethanol content on R_F in 2.5 M NaCl solutions.

A: Neomycin group: —□—□— neomycin A, --●--●-- neomycin B, ·▲···▲· neomycin C.

B: Nebramycin group: --■--■-- apramycin, ···○···○··· kanamycin A, ·-●·-·●-· kanamycin B, —△—△— tobramycin.

(1 mg/ml) were made and 1μl aliquots were spotted. The spray reagent consisted of 0.2g of ninhydrin, 0.5g of p-dimethylaminobenzaldehyde, dissolved in a mixture of 10ml of cyclohexane and 70ml of ethanol.

After pre-drying and spraying, the plates were heated at 105°C for 10 minutes.

For comparison of retention behavior of the studied aminoglycosides in different salt solutions we applied principal component analysis (PCA).[6]

216

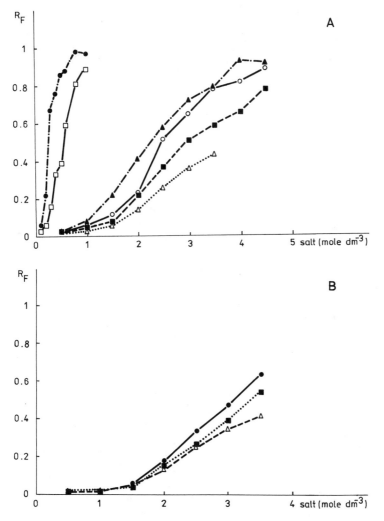

Fig. 2. Effect of salts and their concentrations on R_F of tobramycin.

A: $\cdot-\blacktriangle-\cdot-\blacktriangle-\cdot$ NH_4Cl, $-\!\!\circ\!\!-\!\!\circ\!\!-$ LiCl, $--\blacksquare--\blacksquare--$ NaCl, $-\!\!\square\!\!-\!\!\square\!\!-$ KCl, $\cdot\cdot\triangle\cdot\cdot\cdot\triangle\cdot\cdot$ $MgCl_2$, $-\cdot-\bullet-\cdot-\cdot-\bullet-\cdot$ $CaCl_2$.

B: $-\!\!\bullet\!\!-\!\!\bullet\!\!-$ KI, $\cdot\cdot\cdot\blacksquare\cdot\cdot\cdot\blacksquare\cdot\cdot\cdot$ KBr, $--\triangle--\triangle--$ KCl.

RESULTS AND DISCUSSION

The most important members of aminoglycoside antibiotics are: neomycin A, B and C in the neomycin group and tobramycin, apramycin, kanamycin A and B in the nebramycin family, the structures of which are shown below.

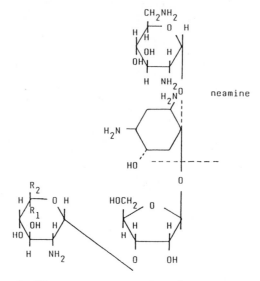

neamine

neomycin B: R_1 = CH_2NH_2 R_2 = H

neomycin C: R_1 = H R_2 = CH_2NH_2

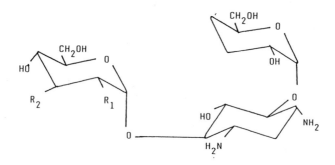

kanamycin B: R_1 = NH_2 R_2 = OH

tobramycin: R_1 = NH_2 R_2 = H

kanamycin A: R_1 = OH R_2 = OH

apramycin

Dependence of the Retention Behavior of Aminoglycosides on the Ethanol Concentration

The effect of ethanol concentration was studied in 2.5 M sodium chloride solutions containing 0 to 40 percent of ethanol. The retention behavior is illustrated in Figure 1.

The retention order of derivatives is identical in each case, in the neomycin group: neomycin C<B<A, in the nebramycin group: kanamycin B<tobramycin<apramycin<kanamycin A.

The highest R_F values were measured in aqueous solutions and practically no effect of ethanol on the retention behavior of the compounds was observed.

Dependence of the Retention Behavior of Aminoglycosides on the Salts

The results obtained with tobramycin are shown in Figure 2. All the studied aminoglycosides behave similarly. The retention order is always the same.

In solutions of univalent cations in the concentration range of 0 to 1-1.5 M compounds do not move from the origin. This is followed by a practically linear range from 1.5 to 3-3.5 M salt concentrations. Above this range the R_F values alter slowly as a function of the salt concentration.

At a given concentration the R_F order of a given compound is: $K^+ < Na^+ < Li^+ < NH_4^+$.

In solutions of divalent cations the aminoglycosides move from the origin at concentrations as low as at 0.1-0.2 M. And this is followed by a sharply rising linear profile and then, at 0.8-1 M concentrations, the curves become slightly flat. R_F order of compounds is: $Mg^{2+} < Ca^{2+}$.

The effect of anions: the R_F - salt concentration curves in solutions of potassium chloride, - bromide and -iodide are similar to those measured in solutions of univalent cations. The R_F values rise in order of $Cl^- < Br^- < I^-$.

Results of Principal Component Analysis (PCA)

For PCA linear correlations were calculated between the corresponding R_M values and the salt concentrations:

$$R_M = ac + b \qquad (1)$$

where R_F is the actual R_M value of an aminoglycoside determined in different salt solutions of concentration c. The PCA eigen value shows that there is a common feature in the effect of salts, this explains their effect at 97.76 percent. The PC loadings prove the same, all the compounds are in the first principal component.

On the basis of their salt - sensitivity (the slope of Equation 1.) the aminoglycosides can be divided into two groups (Figure 3). Apramycin and kanamycin A differ from the other compounds, this is probably due to their more polar structure.

The eluents can also be divided into two groups (Figure 4). There is practically no difference between solutions of univalent cations, but they markedly differ from solutions of divalent cations. This fact may be explained by different hydration energies.[7]

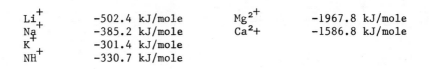

Li^+	-502.4 kJ/mole	Mg^{2+}	-1967.8 kJ/mole
Na^+	-385.2 kJ/mole	Ca^{2+}	-1586.8 kJ/mole
K^+	-301.4 kJ/mole		
NH^+	-330.7 kJ/mole		

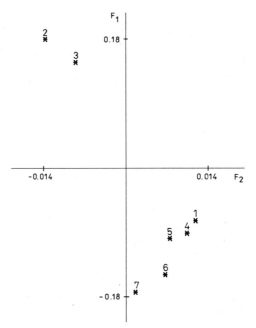

Fig. 3. Two dimensional map of PC loadings. 1 – tobramycin, 2 – apramycin, 3 – kanamycin A, 4 – kanamycin B, 5 – neomycin A, 6 – neomycin B, 7 – neomycin C.

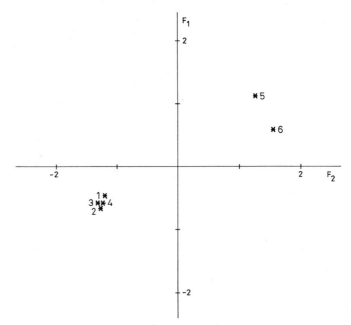

Fig. 4. Two dimensional map of PC variables. 1 – LiCl, 2 – NaCl, 3 – KCl, 4 – NH_4Cl, 5 – $MgCl_2$, 6 – $CaCl_2$.

For divalent ions the basis of separation is mainly adsorption, for univalent ions a mixed mechanism is most likely, however this has not been confirmed unequivocally and further work is necessary. There is no difference between results of TLC and OPLC investigations.

ACKNOWLEDGEMENT

The author thanks to Mr. T. Cserháti for his help in computing of PCA.

REFERENCES

1. Gy. Bacsa, J. Jávor: J.Liq.Chromatogr. 7:2803 (1984).
2. T. Cserháti, B. Bordás and E. Tyihák: J.Chromatogr. 365:289 (1986).
3. E. Tyihák, E. Mincsovics and H. Kalász: J.Chromatogr. 174:75 (1979).
4. E. Mincsovics, E. Tyihák and H. Kalász: J.Chromatogr. 191:293 (1980).
5. E. Tyihák, E. Mincsovics, H. Kalász and J. Nagy: J. Chromatogr. 211:45 (1981).
6. K. V. Mardia, J. T. Kent, and J. M. Billy: Multivariate Analysis, Academic Press, London 1979.
7. G. M. Barrow: Physical Chemistry, McGraw-Hill Book Company, New York, St. Louis, San Francisco, Toronto, London 1961.

A NOTE ON: QUANTITATIVE DETERMINATION OF AMFETAMINIL BY HIGH

PERFORMENCE THIN-LAYER CHROMATOGRAPHY

Bernd Renger

Mundipharma GmbH
D 6250, Limburg, Germany

INTRODUCTION

Amfetaminil (AN 1$^{(R)}$, 2-Phenyl-N-[1'-methyl-2'-phenethyl]-amino-acetonitrile) is a psychotropic substance with a general stimulating effect differing distinctly from that of amphetamine[1-5]. Although an α-amino-nitrile the compound shows remarkable resistance towards hydrolysis in pure water and diluted hydrochloric acid, thus ensuring sufficient stability for its therapeutic application. This stability is a result of the limited solubility of amfetaminil base, as well as its hydrochloride salt, in aqueous media[6,7], and has been proven by using ^{1}H-NMR[8].

The compound is hydrolysed, however, in mixtures of organic solvents and water in the presence of traces of acids and bases[7,8,9] as shown in the following scheme:

This decomposition to amphetamine, benzaldehyde and hydrogen cyanide has been shown to occur during all reported attempts to develop methods for the analysis of amfetaminil by TLC on silica or aluminia[7,10-16] or by GLC[13,15,17]. Pharmacopeia monographs for amfetaminil therefore contain limit tests for benzaldehyde, titratable basic substances and cyanide to ensure the purity of the product, whereas the drug was determined by quantitative hydrolysis followed by titration of the formed cyanide[18]. This method, however, is not applicable to pharmaceutical preparations due to interferences caused by the presence of excipients, while improved modifications of the original assay procedure are somewhat time consuming[19].

To determine the quality of our amfetaminil-containing pharmaceutical preparations, we therefore attempted to develop a suitable chromatographic system, to meet the following criteria:-

1. no decomposition of the compound during chromatography, thus proving its identity, purity and stability.
1. clear separation of potential decomposition products and possibly their quantitative determination
3. no interference with the excipients
4. good reproducibility of the amfetaminil assay
5. simple work up prior to chromatography
6. rapid, simple and efficient chromatographic method

As none of the tested HPLC and GLC methods fit the first two requirements, we concentrated on the use of TLC or HPTLC which are the methods of choice in our laboratories for quality control procedures. The only TLC-system on which amfetaminil was reported to be stable used cellulose plates with a cyclohexane-ethyl acetate mixture as mobile phase[15]. This showed poor reproducibility, and did not separate amfetaminil and benzaldehyde. Testing of different alkyl-modified reversed-phase (RP) TLC plates was unsuccessful due to them being too acidic in nature. Even prewashing the RP-TLC plates with different bases followed by extensive drying did not prevent the decomposition of the amfetaminil on chromatography.

A new cyanopropyl-modified type of HPTLC plate was then tested with excellent results. This type of plate gives a hydrophilic layer with medium polarity which can act either as a RP-phase or a normal phase, depending on the eluent used[20]. As a normal phase with a mobile phase of n-hexane/tert.-butylmethyl-ether (9:1) the cyano-plates showed excellent separation of amfetaminil from its decomposition products (Figure 1).

The slow decomposition of amfetaminil using this system did not affect the assay procedure providing the densitometric evaluation was carried out within 20 minutes after plate development. The calibration function, area versus µg amfetaminil per spot, shows a linear relationship with a limit of detection of about 1µg. (Figure 2).

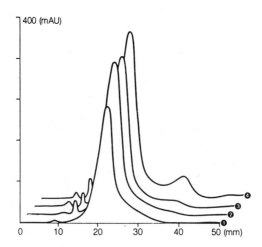

Fig. 1. Thin-layer chromatography on cyanopropyl-modified silica HPTLC plates (Merck). Mobile phase: n-hexane/tert. butyl-methyl-ether 9:1. Track 1: amfetaminil. Track 2: amfetaminil + 1% amphetamine + 1% benzaldehyde. Track 3: amfetaminil + 3% amphetamine + 3% benzaldehyde. Track 4: amfetaminil + 10% amphetamine + 10% benzaldehyde. Detection: in-situ evaluation with scanner (Camag), reflectance UV 260 nm.

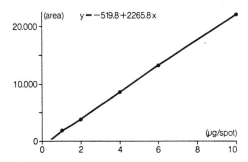

Fig. 2. Densitometry calibration plot of amfetaminil.

This method gave a reproducibility of approximately 3% which indicated that further attempts to increase the accuracy of the procedure by pre- or postconditioning of the plates was unnecessary for our requirements.

The very fast and simple chromatography was complemented by rapid sample preparation. Thus the pulverised tablets were agitated for 30 seconds in an ultrasonic bath with 1ml of tert. butyl-methylether per tablet and then centrifuged for 5 minutes at 10,000 rpm. The 1µl of the clear supernatant solution was spotted onto the HPTLC plate without any further treatment, the validated recovery rate was approximately 97%. No interference with other components of the tablets occured, and the total time required for the amfetaminil assay in pharmaceutical preparations was shortened to approximately 40 minutes.

CONCLUSIONS

This HPTLC method for amfetaminil demonstrates that in certain cases HPTLC can be superior to more sophisticated chromatographic methods such as high performance or gas liquid chromatography. In addition the new types of plate currently being introduced, although seemingly to be quite exotic, can help to solve problems which had appeared to be insoluble.

REFERENCES

1. J. Klosa, J.Prakt.Chemie., 20:275 (1963).
2. D. Krause, Zbl.Pharm., 113:1267 (1974).
3. A. Herbst, Ztschr. ärztl.Fortbildung, 59:670 (1965), 64:38 (1970).
4. R. E. Koch, M. Pambor, K. H. Parnitzke, R. Rabending, Z.inn.Med., 17:122 (1962).
5. H. Teichmann, H. Knaape; Psychiatrie, Neurologie und Psychologie 298 (1970).
6. J. Klosa; Arzneim-Forsch. (Drug Res.) 24:134: (1974) 25, 1252:1863 (1975).
7. T. Beyrich, R. Glöckl, Pharmazie 27:95 (1972), 28:31 (1973).
8. B. Krieg, Arzneim.-Forsch.(Drug Res.) 24:133 (1974), 25:836 (1975).
9. J. Klosa; Dtsch.Apotheker Ztg. 112:423 (1972).
10. G. Bohn, G. Rücker, Arzneim.-Forsch. (Drug Res.) 21:2114 (1974).
11. K. H. Beyer, W. Strassner, D. Klinge, Dtsch.Apotheker Ztg., 111:677 (1971).
12. H. Hoffmann, Dtsch.Apotheker Ztg., 111:680 (1971).
13. K. Besserer, Arzneim.Forsch (Drug Res.) 22: 1737 (1972).
14. B. Salvesen, B. Tetsa and A. H. Beckett, Arzneim.-Forsch.(Drug Res.) 24:137 (1974).
15. H. Honecker, H. Coper, Arzneim.-Forsch.(Drug Res.) 25:442 (1975).

16. K. H. Scholz, Dtsch.Apotheker Ztg., 123:619 (1983).
17. G. Bohn, A. Audick, P. Hoeltzenbein, Z. Rechtsmedizin 79:189 (1977).
18. DAB 7-DDR.
19. B. Unterhalt, Pharm.Ztg., 122:1132 (1977).
20. W. Jost, H. E. Hauck, Proc. 3rd. Intern.Symposium on Instrumental High Performance Thin-Layer Chromatography, Würzburg (1985).

A NOTE ON: A THIN-LAYER CHROMATOGRAPHIC SCREENING METHOD FOR THE TRANQUILLIZERS AZAPERONE, PROPIOPROMAZINE AND CARAZOLOL IN SWINE TISSUES

N. Haagsma, E. R. Bathelt and J. W. Engelsma

Department of the Science of Food of Animal Origin
Section Chemistry, Faculty of Veterinary Medicine
The University of Utrecht, P.O. Box 80 175
NL-3508 TD, Utrecht, The Netherlands

INTRODUCTION

The application of tranquillizers to stressed swine prior to transport may give rise to a residue problem. For the determination of tranquillizer residues in food of animal origin some methods have been described. These include procedures such as gas chromatography (1-3), high-performance liquid chromatography (4, 5), thin-layer chromatography (6) and direct fluorimetry (7). Most of these procedures are directed towards individual tranquillizers (1-3, 5, 6). The need was felt to develop a relatively simple qualitative thin-layer chromatographic (TLC) screening procedure which should determine the neuroleptics azaperone and propiopromazine and the β-blocker carazolol in swine tissue.

The present paper describes such a method using two-dimensional high-performance thin-layer chromatography (HPTLC). For efficient sample clean-up solid-phase extraction (SPE) was used.

EXPERIMENTAL

The ground tissue was heated with a 1 mol l^{-1} sodium hydroxide solution at 95°C and extracted with ethyl ether. After addition of petroleum ether the solution was cleaned up and concentrated with the aid of a silica gel solid phase extraction column. Elution was performed by means of methanol containing hydrochloric acid. Identification was performed by two-dimensional HPTLC on aluminium backed sheets (silica gel 60, F254, 5 x 5 cm), using the solvent system: dichloromethane-acetone-ammonia 25% (100:100:5 v/v) in direction a (viz. Figure 1) and n-butanol-acetic acid-water (80:20:100 v/v, organic layer (8)) in direction b (viz. Figure 1). The plate was then examined under 254 nm UV light for dark-blue spots of azaperone and azaperol and the brown spot of carazolol on a greenish fluorescent background and under UV light at 366 nm for the propiopromazine spot. At this wavelength the propiopromazine sulphoxide can also be observed.

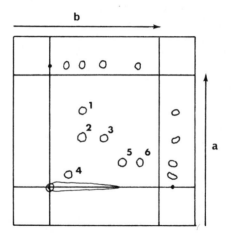

Fig. 1.   Thin-layer chromatogram of tissue extract.   For chromatographic
conditions, viz. text. a = direction of first development;
b = direction of second development. 1 = azaperone, 2 = azaperol,
3 = propiopromazine, 4 = propiopromazine sulphoxide, 5 = matrix
compound (kidney), 6 = carazolol.

Results and Discussions

A characteristic TLC chromatogram is shown in Figure 1.   Metabolites
such as azaperol (3) and propiopromazine sulfoxide (2) are also separated
and detected.

The eluent (1), used for the first development does not separate
carazolol from propiopromazine sulfoxide.   However, separation from nearly
all matrix components is achieved, as these remain at the origin.   The
second development completes the separation.   It was observed that, in this
second development, carazolol was separated from a minor matrix compound
which was found to be only in samples from kidney.

In spiked tissues, the presence of concentrations down to 125 µg kg^{-1}
for carazolol, 50µg kg^{-1} for azaperone and 25 µg kg^{-1} for propiopromazine
can be demonstrated in this way.   For kidney tissue these detection levels
are sufficient for azaperone and propiopromazine, but not for carazolol.
However, the sensitivity for carazolol is sufficient when injection sites
are examined.   In an experiment with swine treated with the usual doses the
presence of propiopromazine and azaperol could be established in kidney
tissue 8 h after administration, whilst at the injection sites all three
tranquillizers could be detected.   More detailed information will be
published in due course[9].

Acknowledgements

This study was supported by the Veterinary Hygiene Public Health
Inspectorate.   The authors thank Drs. G. T. W. van der Meer, R. V. V.,
District 8, for providing the tissues of swine treated with tranquillizers.

REFERENCES

1.   W. Arneth, Fleischwirtsch., 65:945 (1985).
2.   W. Arneth, Fleischwirtsch., 66:922 (1986).

3. A. G. Rauws, M. Olling, J. Freudenthal and M. ten Ham, Tox.Appl. Pharmacol., 35:333 (1976).
4. R. Etter, R. Battaglia, J. Noser and F. Schuppisser, Mitt.Geb. Lebensm.Hyg., 75:447 (1984).
5. B. Hoffmann, H. A. Meemken and W. Groebel, Lebensmittelch. u. Gerichtl. Chemie, 36:104 (1982).
6. M. Olling, R. W. Stephany and A. G. Rauws, J.Vet.Pharmacol.Therap., 4:291 (1981).
7. J. W. Engelsma and J. Simons, Vet.Quart., 7:73 (1985).
8. Anon. Prüfungsvorschrift für Injektionslösung (Suacron) für Tiere, Boehringer Mannheim, 1978.
9. N. Haagsma, E. R. Bathelt and J. W. Engelsma, J.Chromatogr., accepted for publication.

A NOTE ON: A SIMPLE AND RAPID HIGH PERFORMANCE THIN-LAYER CHROMATOGRAPHIC
METHOD FOR THE SEPARATION AND IDENTIFICATION OF HEAVY METAL
DITHIOCARBAMATES AND RELATED COMPOUNDS

J. E. Futter

Robinson Brothers Limited
West Bromwich
West Midlands B70 0AH, UK

INTRODUCTION

Dithiocarbamates and other accelerators such as thiuram sulphides
(thiurams), are widely used in the Rubber Industry for the curing of
natural and synthetic rubber, as stabilisers against ultra-violet radiation, and as heat-ageing inhibitors (antioxidants). Analytical methods
for these compounds have been reviewed by Burger[1] and Auler[2], the
latter giving special emphasis to paper chromatographic methods. Prior to
1965 very few applications of thin-layer chromatography (TLC) were reported
in this field. However, in 1969 Kreiner and Warner[3] published detailed
methods for the identification of many rubber compounding ingredients by
TLC using plates self-coated with Merck Silica Gel G (Non-fluorescent).
The visualization procedures employed by these workers were complex. In
1970 Rai and Kukreja[4] published a short paper on the separation of the
diethyl dithiocarbamates of bismuth, cobalt, copper, chromium lead, mercury, nickel, palladium, silver, thallium and uranium, using very simple
eluents and the same adsorbent. Compounds were detected by their own color
or visualized using yellow ammonium sulphide. Solution strengths and
application volumes were not reported. Onuska[5] quantitatively determined
various N,N-dialkyldithiocarbamates and thiurams in waste waters using
Eastman pre-coated 6060 silica gel fluorescent plates and a densitometer.
Samples were solvent extracted with chloroform, pre-concentrated on an
evaporator then converted into the copper complexes prior to chromatography
and quantitation. Rao and Chopra[6] separated dithiocarbamates, xanthates
and thioxanthates of cobalt, nickel, palladium, molybdenum, lead and bismuth on Silica Gel G layers. Individual spots on preparative plates were
extracted with chloroform and quantified spectrophotometrically.

The present method, using high performance (HP) TLC, is simple and
rapid, with very low detection limits in the range 10-500ng.

EXPERIMENTAL

Analytical grade solvents and reagents supplied by BDH Chemicals Ltd.
were used. Samples of dithiocarbanates (DTC's) and thiurams of normal
commercial quality were supplied by Robinson Brothers Ltd. ex works. The
dithiocarbamates (DTC's) were used without purification. Thiurams were
recrystallized from hot water/ethanol mixtures except for tetrabutylthiuram

disulphide. The latter is an oil at ambient temperature and proved
difficult to purify. It was therefore used as supplied. Chlorinated
solvents of the lowest possible polarity, compatible with solubility, were
used in order to minimize initial spot sizes (Table 1). Solution strengths
were 0.1% m/v and 0.01% m/v.

Plates

10 x 10 cm Merck Silica Gel 60 HPTLC plates, Cat. Nos. 5628 and 5631
(Non-fluorescent), were used without activation.

Samples were spaced 10mm from the lower edge with spots 5mm apart. A
Camag Nanomat II applicator with Drummond disposable micropipettes, (0.5,
1 µl), or a Hamilton 1 µl syringe Model 7101, (for 0.1, 0.2 µl applications), were used. Loadings were thus 10 - 1000ng. Twin through tanks,
(Camag 25155), with wick, were used for vapor phase equilibration (30 mins)
and elution. For the composite dithiocarbamate plate (Figure 1) maximum
separation was achieved by eluting over 8cms. Elution times were short –
typically 10 to 15 mins – a reflection of low eluent polarities.

Eluent Systems

To minimize gradient elution effects complex solvent mixtures were
avoided. The final choices were:-

(a) chloroform – cyclohexane – toluene (1:1:1) v/v – for dithiocarbamates
(b) toluene – ethyl acetate (10:1) v/v – for thiuram sulphides
R_f and R_{st} values are shown in Table 2.

Table 1. Accelerator Solvents and Detection Limits (Approximate)

Accelerator		Solvent	Detection limits (ng)		
			NaN_3-I_2	Dithizone/ NH_3*	$CuSO_4$	F_{254}
Cupric dimethyl DTC (CuDD)	A	10	50	–	20
Cupric diethyl DTC (CuED)	A	10	10	–	10
Cupric dibutyl DTC (CuBuD)	B	10	50	–	10
Cupric pentamethylene DTC (CuPD)	A	10	50	–	200
Nickel dimethyl DTC (NiDD)	C	10	500	50	200
Nickel diethyl DTC (NiDC)	A	10	100	50	100
Nickel dibutyl DTC (NiBuD)	B	10	100	50	100
Nickel pentamethylene DTC (NiPD)	A	10	100	50	100
Zinc dimethyl DTC (ZMD)	A	20	100	200	50
Zinc diethyl DTC (ZDC)	A	20	100	200	50
Zinc dibutyl DTC (ZBuD)	B	20	100	200	50
Zinc pentamethylene DTC (ZPD)	A	20	100	200	50
Tetramethylthiuram MS (TMS)	A	<10	–	100	10
Tetramethylthiuram DS (TMT)	A	<10	–	100	10
Tetraethylthiuram DS (TET)	A	<10	–	100	10
Tetrabutylthiuram DS (TBuT)	A	10	–	100	50
Pentamethylene MS (PTM)	A	10	–	200	50
Pentamethylene DS (PTD)	A	10	–	200	50

Key: DTC = dithiocarbamate; MS = monosulphide; DS = disulphide
       (A) = chloroform, (B) = carbon tetrachloride,
       (C) = 1,1,2,2,- tetrachloroethane
       *Non-fluorescent plate

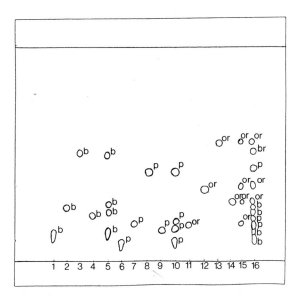

Fig. 1.   Separation of N,N-Dialkyl Dithiocarbamates. Merck 5631 HPTLC
plate. Eluent System (A). 8 cm elution distance. Elution time
12 minutes. Detection – Reagent 2). Loading 500 ng.   1 = CuDD;
2 = CuED; 3 = CuBuD; 4 = CuPD; 5 = Cu (Composite); 6 = NiDD;
7 = NiDC; 8 = NiBuD; 9 = NiPD; 10 = Ni (Composite); 11 = ZMD;
12 = ZDC; 13 = ZBuD; 14 = ZPD; 15 = Zn (Composite); 16 = All.

Table 2. R_f and R_{st} Values of N,N – Dialkyl Dithiocarbamates and Thiurams

Dithio-carbamate	CuDD	CuED	CuBuD	CuPD	NiDD	NiCD	NiBuD	NiPD	ZMD	ZDC	ZBuD	ZPD
R_f X 100	12.4	25.2	50.4	19.5	8.0	17.7	41.6	14.6	16.8	33.3	55.8	27.9
R_{st} X 100	22.2	45.2	90.3	34.9	14.3	31.7	74.6	26.2	30.1	59.7	100	50.0

Thiuram	TMS	TMT	TET	TBuT	PTM	PTD
R_f X 100	21.5	36.5	49.5	66.0	39.5	50.0
R_{st} X 100	32.6	55.3	75.0	100	59.8	75.8

R_{st} = $\dfrac{\text{distance from starting point to center of substance}}{\text{distance from starting point to center of STANDARD}}$

Standards:-   ZBuD for dithiocarbamates
TBuT for thiurams

Chromogenic Spray Reagents

1.   "Iodine Azide". Dissolve 3g sodium azide in 100mls 0.05M iodine
aqueous solution. Bivalent sulphur compounds decolorize the reagent, white
spots thus appearing against a brown iodine-stained background. Low
levels, which may appear after 30 to 60 seconds delay are masked by

excessive spraying. Pre-spraying with starch solution results in a black background and enhanced contrast at high sample loadings but spots in the 10ng to 50ng range are partially obscured. This modification is best avoided.

2. Dithizone/ammonia. (For dithiocarbamates only)
(i) Spray non-fluorescent plates with 0.05% m/v dithizone in carbon tet-rachloride.
(ii) Lower the plate into a tank containing ammonia vapor, (ex 0.880 sp.gr. solution), for 30 seconds.

The green background is bleached to pale yellow and colored spots of varying intensities appear.

Cupric DTC's - intense brown; Nickel DTC's - purple; Zinc DTC's - pale pink.

(Fluorescent plates give an intense red background, masking most spots, and must be avoided.)

3. Copper (II) Sulphate. Dissolve 10g of the pentahydrate in 100mls of water. Nickel DTC' (at low "invisible" loadings) - brown spots. Zinc DTC' - brown spots. Thiuram sulphides (selected) - brown-yellow spots.

RESULTS AND DISCUSSION

Separation of accelerators within an homologous series was easily achieved. R_f values were inversely related to molecular polarities. A second elution was helpful in enhancing separation of the pentamethylene-based accelerators from adjacent compounds, enabling positive identifications to be made. The characteristic colors given by the dithiocarba-

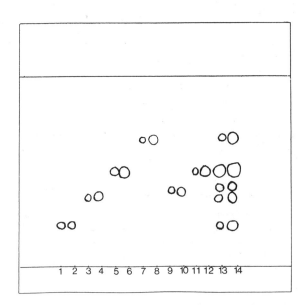

Fig. 2. Separation of Thiuram Sulphides. Merck 5628 HPTLC plate. Eluent System (B). 7 cm elution distance. Elution time 11 minutes. Detection - (a). UV Fluorescence 254 nm. (b) Reagent (1). Loading -5, 10 ng. 1,2 = TMS; 3,4 = TMT; 5,6 TET; 7,8 TBuT; 9,10 = PTM; 11,12 = PTD; 13,14 = All.

mates when sprayed with the dithizone/ammonia reagent assisted in identifying the chelated metals, even when originally present at very low, nonvisible, loadings. Iodine azide may, in this particular case, be applied to the plate subsequently, giving immediate distinction between DTC's and thiurams, should the former be absent (figure 2). The brown spots given by copper (II) sulphate spray were helpful for visualizing zinc dithiocarbamates, (distinction from dithizone/ammonia), and low levels of the nickel equivalents.

Detection limits were low for all visualization techniques, with limit inversely related to elution distance. Over short distances as little as 5ng is detectable for thiurams using "iodine-azide" reagent. This remains one of the most sensitive of all chromogenic reagents for the qualitative evaluation of bivalent sulphur compounds. Unfortunately its lack of selectivity makes R_F matching against known accelerator standards essential.

The main advantages of the current methodology employing HPTLC compared to conventional thin-layer chromatography are lower detection limits, excellent separation over shorter distances, better reproducibility and, most significantly, speed. A combination of the above mentioned elution and detection techniques enables positive assignments for most of the accelerators present in a sample to be made easily, with minimum plate usage.

ACKNOWLEDGEMENT

The author is grateful to the directors of Robinson Brothers Limited for permission to publish this work.

REFERENCES

1. V. L. Burger, Rubber Chem.Technol., 32:1452 (1959).
2. H. Auler, Gummi Asbest Kunststoffe, 14: 1024, 1081, (1960).
3. J. G. Kreiner and W. C. Warner J.Chromatog., 44:315 (1969).
4. J. Rai and V. P. Kukreja, Chromatographia, 3:41 (1970).
5. F. I. Onuska, Anal.Lett., 7:327 (1974).
6. A. L. J. Rao and S. Chopra, J.Inst.Chemists (India), 57:197 (1985).

COMPOUND INDEX